Fibromyalgia

T0271995

Fibromyalgia

Edited by

Bill H. McCarberg
Kaiser Permanente and University of California
San Diego, California, USA

Daniel J. Clauw
The University of Michigan
Ann Arbor, Michigan, USA

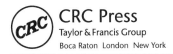

CRC Press
Taylor & Francis Group
Boca Raton London New York

CRC Press is an imprint of the
Taylor & Francis Group, an **informa** business

CRC Press
Taylor & Francis Group
6000 Broken Sound Parkway NW, Suite 300
Boca Raton, FL 33487-2742

First issued in paperback 2017

© 2009 by Taylor & Francis Group, LLC
CRC Press is an imprint of Taylor & Francis Group, an Informa business

No claim to original U.S. Government works
ISBN-13: 978-1-4200-8679-9 (hbk)
ISBN-13: 978-1-138-11291-9 (pbk)

Library of Congress Cataloging-in-Publication Data

Fibromyalgia / edited by Bill H. McCarberg, Daniel J. Clauw.
    p. ; cm.
    Includes bibliographical references and index.
    ISBN-13: 978-1-4200-8679-9 (hardcover : alk. paper)
    ISBN-10: 1-4200-8679-0 (hardcover : alk. paper) 1. Fibromyalgia—
Treatment. I. McCarberg, Bill H. II. Clauw, Daniel J.
    [DNLM: 1. Fibromyalgia—therapy. 2. Fibromyalgia—diagnosis. WE
544 F4412 2009]
    RC927.3.F48 2009
    616.7'42—dc22

                                                            2009017626

Visit the Taylor & Francis Web site at
http://www.taylorandfrancis.com

and the CRC Press Web site at
http://www.crcpress.com

Preface

Fibromyalgia (FM) presents a challenge to health care providers. A heterogeneous condition with uncertain pathophysiology has led to a persistent debate within the medical community regarding FM's nature and validity. FM is underdiagnosed and suboptimally treated with research indicating that patients seeking medical care face multiple barriers. In one investigation involving 76 patients ≥60 years presenting for a general geriatric clinic visit, only 1 of 25 patients identified with "probable fibromyalgia" had been previously diagnosed (1). Most patients experience FM symptoms for five to seven years and many consult with multiple physicians prior to diagnosis (2).

FM has received a great deal of attention over the past two decades. Despite the interest in this syndrome, it lacks a clear consensus as to how best to treat patients who meet the diagnostic criteria, and currently there is no known cure. This set of factors makes interactions with patients and successful treatment difficult and demanding. However, FM is recognized as a legitimate clinical entity, and the presence or absence of physician support is likely to exert a strong positive or negative impact on the health of the suffering individuals.

FM consists of many conditions with countless presentations. Scientists are only now beginning to define and analyze its complex biomedical and psychological mechanisms.

In this text, we present a logical flow to assist the primary care provider in his or her encounter with FM patients. Most providers attempt to arrive at a diagnosis through recognition of patterns of symptoms. The various presentations are described with an explanation of why these may differ in patients. The etiology of FM is not fully elucidated but current advances with recent functional MRI findings are described.

Once diagnosed, patients are interested in disease progression. The natural history and pathophysiology of the disease are described in detail. The evaluation of the patient includes diseases that can mimic FM. Treatment including nonpharmacologic, complementary, and alternative therapy, and the most recent pharmacologic options and investigational drugs are described.

The most perplexing and difficult issues for the clinicians are psychosocial comorbidities, disability, exercise, and how to motivate the patient to change behavior. All these topics are examined in detail as stand alone articles relevant to the patient encounters occurring frequently in the office.

This book is designed for the primary care provider. The majority of FM patients will present to primary care, receive most treatment in primary care, and even if referred, will likely return to primary care for ongoing management. The primary care provider is best equipped to deal with all the concerns of the FM patient. FM is like many other chronic conditions: it has no cure, quality of life is significantly impaired, patient self-efficacy and acceptance is key to good outcomes, and a caring empathetic provider results in patients who learn to cope despite challenges.

This text is essential reading for the primary provider. Even if one doubts the validity of FM, patients still need evaluation, treatment, hope, and a caring provider. The latest science is important for best outcomes. An approach to the FM patient and treatment options are critical for improved quality of life. We all must accept the challenge of improving the pain and dysfunction in our patients. Presented here is a new approach with valuable guidance to enhance our practice skills in a condition affecting countless numbers of patients.

Bill H. McCarberg
Daniel J. Clauw

REFERENCES

1. Gowin KM. Diffuse pain syndromes in the elderly. Rheum Dis Clin North Am 2000; 26:(3):673–682.
2. Goldenberg DL. Fibromyalgia syndrome a decade later: what have we learned? Arch Intern Med 1999; 159:777–785.

Contents

Contributors

Robert Alan Bonakdar Scripps Center for Integrative Medicine, Scripps Clinic, La Jolla, California, U.S.A.

Lesley M. Arnold Department of Psychiatry, Women's Health Research Program, University of Cincinnati College of Medicine, Cincinnati, Ohio, U.S.A.

Daniel J. Clauw Division of Rheumatology, The University of Michigan, Ann Arbor, Michigan, U.S.A.

Leslie J. Crofford Division of Rheumatology and Women's Health, and Center for the Advancement of Women's Health, University of Kentucky, Lexington, Kentucky, U.S.A.

A. deHueck Physiotherapy Department, Joseph Brant Memorial Hospital, Burlington, Ontario, Canada

Vikrum Figoora Department of Neurology and Psychiatry, Saint Louis University School of Medicine, St. Louis, Missouri, U.S.A.

S. E. Gowans Allied Health, University Health Network; Department of Physical Therapy, University of Toronto, Toronto, Ontario, Canada

Marissa L. Marshak Clinical Social Worker, Ann Arbor, Michigan, U.S.A.

Bill H. McCarberg Chronic Pain Management Program, Kaiser Permanente San Diego, and University of California, San Diego, California, U.S.A.

Raymond C. Tait Department of Neurology and Psychiatry, Saint Louis University School of Medicine, St. Louis, Missouri, U.S.A.

Dennis C. Turk Department of Anesthesiology, University of Washington, Seattle, Washington, U.S.A.

David A. Williams Chronic Pain and Fatigue Research Center, and Department of Anesthesiology, Medicine, Psychiatry, and Psychology, University of Michigan, Ann Arbor, Michigan, U.S.A.

Hilary D. Wilson Department of Anesthesiology, University of Washington, Seattle, Washington, U.S.A.

1 Etiology of Fibromyalgia

Daniel J. Clauw

Division of Rheumatology, The University of Michigan, Ann Arbor, Michigan, U.S.A.

INTRODUCTION

Clinical practitioners commonly see patients with pain and other somatic symptoms that they cannot adequately explain on the basis of the degree of damage or inflammation noted in peripheral tissues. In fact, this may be among the most common predicament that individuals seek medical attention for (1). Typically, an evaluation is performed looking for a "cause" for the pain. If none is found, these individuals are often given a diagnostic label that merely connotes that the patient has chronic pain in a region of the body, without an underlying mechanistic cause [e.g., chronic low back pain, headache, temporomandibular disorder (TMD), etc.]. In other cases, the label given alludes to an underlying mechanism that may or may not be responsible for the individual's pain (e.g., "facet syndrome").

Fibromyalgia (FM) is merely a term used currently for individuals with chronic widespread musculoskeletal pain for which no alternative cause can be identified. Gastroenterologists often see patients with same symptoms and focus on their gastroenterological complaints; they often use the terms functional gastrointestinal (GI) disorder, irritable bowel syndrome (IBS), nonulcer dyspepsia, or esophageal dysmotility to explain the patient's symptoms (2). Neurologists see these patients for their headaches and/or unexplained facial pain, urologists for pelvic pain and urinary symptoms (and use labels such as interstitial cystitis, chronic prostatitis, vulvodynia, and vulvar vestibulitis), dentists for TMD, and so on.

Until recently these unexplained pain syndromes perplexed researchers, clinicians, and patients. However, it is now clear that

- Individuals will sometimes only have one of these "idiopathic" pain syndromes over the course of their lifetime. But more often, individuals with one of these entities, and their family members, are likely to have several of these conditions (3,4). Many terms have been used to describe these coaggregating syndromes and symptoms, including functional somatic syndromes, somatization disorders, allied spectrum conditions, chronic multisymptom illnesses, medically unexplained symptoms, etc. (3,5–7).
- Women are more likely to have these disorders than men, but the sex difference is much more apparent in clinical samples (especially tertiary care) than in population-based samples (8,9).
- Groups of individuals with these conditions (e.g., FM, IBS, headache, TMD, etc.) display diffuse hyperalgesia (increased pain to normally painful stimuli) and/or allodynia (pain to normally nonpainful stimuli) (10–14). This suggests that these individuals have a fundamental problem with pain or sensory processing rather than an abnormality confined to the region of the body where the person is currently experiencing pain.

- Similar types of therapies are efficacious for all of these conditions, including both pharmacological (e.g., tricyclic compounds such as amitriptyline) and nonpharmacological treatments (e.g., exercise, cognitive behavioral therapy). Conversely, individuals with these conditions typically do not respond to therapies that are effective when pain is due to damage or inflammation of tissues [e.g., nonsteroidal anti-inflammatory drugs (NSAIDs), opioids, injections, surgical procedures].

Until perhaps a decade or ago, these conditions were all on somewhat equal (and tenuous) scientific ground. But within a relatively short period of time, research methods such as experimental pain testing, functional imaging, and genetics have led to tremendous advances in the understanding of several of these conditions, most notably FM, IBS, and TMD. Many in the pain field now feel that chronic pain itself is a "disease" and that many of the underlying mechanisms operative in these heretofore-considered idiopathic or "functional" pain syndromes may be similar no matter whether that pain is present throughout the body (e.g., in FM) or is localized to the lower back, the bowel, or the bladder. Because of this, the more contemporary terms used to describe conditions such as FM, IBS, TMD, vulvodynia, and many other entities include "central pain," "neuropathic pain" (when this term is used in this setting, it is meant to imply that the pain is coming from the nervous system rather than the periphery, rather than connoting that the pain is due to nerve damage), or "nonnociceptive pain" (15,16).

The review regarding FM below focuses on our current understanding of this disorder as one of the prototypical "central pain syndromes."

HISTORICAL PERSPECTIVE

Although the term "fibromyalgia" is relatively new, this condition has been described in the medical literature for centuries. Sir William Gowers coined the term "fibrositis" in 1904. During the next half century, fibrositis (as it was then called) was considered by some to be a common cause of muscular pain, by others to be a manifestation of "tension" or "psychogenic rheumatism," and by the rheumatology community, in general, to be a nonentity.

The current concept of FM was established by Smythe and Moldofsky in the mid-1970s (17). The name change reflected an increasing evidence that there was no –*itis* (inflammation) in the connective tissues of individuals with this condition, but instead –*algia* (pain). These authors characterized the most common tender points (regions of extreme tenderness in these individuals), and reported that patients with FM had disturbances in deep and restorative sleep, and that selective stage-4 interruptions induced the symptoms of FM (18). Yunus and others then reported on the major clinical manifestations of patients with FM seen in rheumatology clinics (19).

The next advance in FM was the development of the American College of Rheumatology (ACR) criteria for FM, which were published in 1990 (20). These classification criteria require that an individual have both a history of chronic widespread pain (CWP) and the finding of 11 or more of a possible 18 tender points on examination. These ACR classification criteria were intended for research use to standardize definitions of FM. In this regard, the criteria have been extremely valuable. Unfortunately, many practitioners use these criteria in routine clinical practice to diagnose individual patients; this unintended use has led to many of the current misconceptions regarding FM, which are discussed below.

The finding of diffusely increased tenderness, as well as a lack of finding – itis in the muscles or other tissues of FM patients, led to the change in the name of this entity from fibrositis to FM. The diffuse nature of the pain and tenderness also led many groups of investigators to explore neural mechanisms to explain the underlying pathogenesis of these disorders (21,22). In fact, major advances have only occurred in understanding individual syndromes within this spectrum once investigators concluded that this was not a condition caused by peripheral damage or inflammation, and began to explore central, neural mechanisms of these diseases. Thus, the conditions we now understand best within this spectrum include FM, IBS (previously termed "spastic colitis" until the recognition that there was little –itis and that motility changes were not the major pathological feature), and TMD (previously termed temporomandibular joint disorder until it was recognized that the problem was not largely within the joint).

Fibromyalgia

The ACR criteria for FM require that an individual have both a history of CWP and the finding of 11 or more of 18 possible tender points on examination. Tender points represent nine paired predefined regions of the body, often over musculotendinous insertions (20). If an individual reports pain when a region is palpated with 4 kg of pressure, this is considered a positive tender point. Between 25% and 50% of individuals who have CWP will also have 11 or more tender points, and thus meet criteria for FM (23,24). The prevalence of FM is just as high in rural or nonindustrialized societies as it is in countries such as the United States (25–27).

Significance of Tender Points

At the time the ACR criteria were published it was thought that there may be some unique significance of the locations of tender points. In fact, a term "control points" was coined to describe areas of the body that should not be tender in FM, and individuals were assumed to have a psychological cause for their pain if they were tender in these regions. Since then, we have learned that the tenderness in FM extends throughout the entire body. Thus, relative to the pain threshold that a normal non-FM patient would experience at the same points, "control" regions of the body such as the thumbnail and forehead are just as tender as in FM tender points (28–30). Thus, to assess tenderness in clinical practice, the practitioner can apply pressure wherever he or she wishes. As long as he or she performs this exam with the same pressure in a series of patients, he or she can get a good sense of the overall pain threshold of any individual patient.

The tender point requirement in the ACR criteria not only misrepresents the nature of the tenderness in this condition (i.e., local rather than widespread), but also strongly influences the demographic and psychological characteristics of FM. Women are only 1.5 times more likely than men to experience CWP, but are 10 times more likely than men to have 11 or more tender points (31). Because of this, women are approximately 10 times more likely to meet ACR criteria for FM than men. Yet, most of the men in the population that have CWP but are not tender enough to meet criteria for FM likely have the same underlying problem as the women who meet the ACR criteria for FM.

Another unintended consequence of requiring both CWP and at least 11 tender points to be diagnosed with FM is that many individuals with FM will have high levels of distress. Wolfe has described tender points as a "sedimentation rate for distress" because of population-based studies showing that tender points are more common in distressed individuals (32).

In summary, although many clinicians uniquely associate FM with women who display high levels of distress, much of this is an artifact of: (*i*) the ACR criteria that require 11 tender points and (*ii*) the fact that most studies of FM have originated from clinical samples from tertiary care centers, where healthcare seeking behaviors lead to the fact that psychological and psychiatric comorbidities are much higher (9). When all these biases are eliminated by examining CWP in population-based studies, a clearer picture of FM can be seen and CWP becomes much like chronic musculoskeletal pain in any other region of the body.

ETIOLOGY
Genetic Factors
Research has indicated a strong familial component to the development of FM. First-degree relatives of individuals with FM display an eightfold greater risk of developing FM than those in the general population (4). These studies also show that family members of individuals with FM are much more tender than the family members of controls, regardless of whether they have pain or not. Family members of FM patients are also much more likely to have IBS, TMD, headaches, and a host of other regional pain syndromes (3,33,34). This familial and personal coaggregation of conditions that includes FM was originally collectively termed *affective spectrum disorder* (35) and more recently *central sensitivity syndrome* and chronic multisymptom illness (7,36). In population-based studies, the key symptoms that often coaggregate besides pain are fatigue, memory difficulties, and mood disturbances (7,37). Twin studies suggest that approximately half of the risk of developing CWP is due to genetic factors and the other half due to environmental factors (38).

Recent studies have begun to identify specific genetic polymorphisms that are associated with a higher risk of developing FM. To date, the serotonin 5-HT2A receptor polymorphism T/T phenotype, serotonin transporter, dopamine 4 receptor, and COMT (catecholamine *o*-methyl transferase) polymorphisms have all been noted to be seen in higher frequency in FM (39–42). Note that all of the polymorphisms identified to date involve the metabolism or transport of monoamines, compounds that play a critical role in activity of the human stress response. It is likely that there are scores of genetic polymorphisms, involving other neuromodulators as well as monoamines, which in part determine an individuals' "set point" for pain and sensory processing.

Environmental Factors
As with most illnesses that may have a genetic underpinning, environmental factors may play a prominent role in triggering the development of FM and related conditions. Environmental "stressors" temporally associated with the development of either FM or chronic fatigue syndrome include physical trauma

(especially involving the trunk), certain infections such as Hepatitis C, Epstein-Barr virus, parvovirus, Lyme disease, and emotional stress. The disorder is also associated with other regional pain conditions or autoimmune disorders (22,43,44) (Figs. 1 and 2). Of note, each of these stressors only leads to CWP or FM in approximately 5% to 10% of individuals who are exposed; the overwhelming majority of individuals who experience these same infections or other stressful events regain their baseline state of health.

An excellent recent example of how illnesses such as FM might be triggered occurred in the setting of the deployment of troops to liberate Kuwait

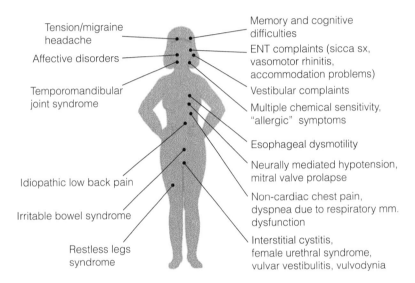

Tension/migraine headache
Affective disorders
Temporomandibular joint syndrome
Idiopathic low back pain
Irritable bowel syndrome
Restless legs syndrome

Memory and cognitive difficulties
ENT complaints (sicca sx, vasomotor rhinitis, accommodation problems)
Vestibular complaints
Multiple chemical sensitivity, "allergic" symptoms
Esophageal dysmotility
Neurally mediated hypotension, mitral valve prolapse
Non-cardiac chest pain, dyspnea due to respiratory mm. dysfunction
Interstitial cystitis, female urethral syndrome, vulvar vestibulitis, vulvodynia

FIGURE 1 Regional or localized syndromes that overlap with fibromyalgia in prevalence, mechanisms, and treatment.

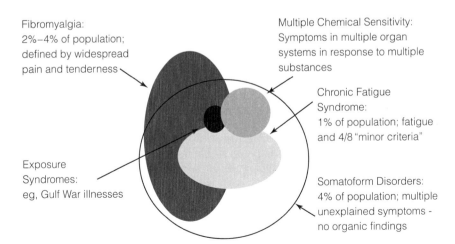

Fibromyalgia:
2%–4% of population; defined by widespread pain and tenderness

Multiple Chemical Sensitivity:
Symptoms in multiple organ systems in response to multiple substances

Chronic Fatigue Syndrome:
1% of population; fatigue and 4/8 "minor criteria"

Exposure Syndromes:
eg, Gulf War illnesses

Somatoform Disorders:
4% of population; multiple unexplained symptoms - no organic findings

FIGURE 2 The "systemic" conditions that overlap with fibromyalgia.

during the Gulf War in 1990 and 1991. The term "Gulf War illnesses" is now commonly used to refer to a constellation of symptoms developed by some 10% to 15% of the 700,000 U.S. troops deployed to the Persian Gulf in the early 1990s. The symptoms, which include headaches, muscle and joint pain, fatigue, memory disorders, and GI distress (7), were seen in troops deployed from the United Kingdom and other countries as well (45). The panels of experts who examined potential causes for these symptoms and syndromes found that the sickness could not be traced to any single environmental trigger, and noted the similarities between these individuals and those diagnosed with FM and chronic fatigue. Furthermore, similar syndromes involving multiple somatic symptoms have been noted in veterans of every war the United States or United Kingdom has been involved in during the past century (46). This suggests that war may be an environment where individuals are simultaneously exposed to a multitude of stressors, triggering the development of this type of illness in susceptible individuals (47).

The above-noted relationship between individuals with other chronic rheumatic or autoimmune disorders deserves special attention because of the relevance to practicing clinicians. As many as 25% of patients correctly diagnosed with generalized inflammatory disorders such as systemic lupus erythematosus (SLE), rheumatoid arthritis (RA), and ankylosing spondylitis will also fulfill ACR criteria for FM (48). However, in clinical practice this coexpression may go unrecognized, especially when the FM develops after the autoimmune disorder or regional pain syndrome. In this setting when comorbid FM goes unrecognized, patients are often unnecessarily treated more aggressively with toxic immunosuppressive drugs.

PATHOGENESIS
Role of Stressors
Once FM develops, the mechanisms responsible for ongoing symptom expression are likely complex and multifactorial. Because of the fact that disparate stressors can trigger the development of these conditions, the human stress response has been closely examined for a causative role. The human stress response is mediated primarily by the activity of the corticotropin-releasing hormone (CRH) nervous system located in the hypothalamus and locus-coeruleus-norepinephrine/autonomic (sympathetic/LC-NE) nervous system located in the brain stem. Recent research suggests that although this system in humans has been highly adaptive throughout history, the stress response may be inappropriately triggered by a wide assortment of everyday occurrences that do not pose a real threat to survival, thus initiating the cascade of physiological responses more frequently than can be tolerated (49).

The type of stress and the environment in which it occurs also have an impact on how the stress response is expressed. It has been noted that victims of accidents experience a higher frequency of FM and myofascial pain than those who cause them, which is congruent with animal studies showing that the strongest physiological responses are triggered by events accompanied by a lack of control or support, and thus perceived as inescapable or unavoidable (50). In humans, daily "hassles" and personally relevant stressors seem to be more capable of causing symptoms than major catastrophic events that do not personally impact on the individual (51).

Two studies performed in the United States just before and after the terrorist attacks of 9/11 point out that not all psychological stress are capable of triggering or exacerbating FM or somatic symptoms. In one study performed by Raphael and colleagues, no difference in pain complaints or other somatic symptoms was seen in residents of New York and New Jersey who had been surveyed prior to 9/11, and then just following the terrorist attacks on the World Trade Center (52). In another study performed in the Washington D.C. region (near the Pentagon—he other site of attack) during the same time period, patients with FM had no worsening of pain or other somatic symptoms following the attacks, compared to just before the attack (53).

Recent reviews regarding the role that stressors (e.g., infections, physical trauma, emotional stress) or catastrophic events may have in triggering the development of FM or related conditions have identified a number of factors that may be much more important than the intensity of the stressor in predicting adverse health outcomes. Female gender, worry or expectation of chronicity, and inactivity or time off work following the stressor make it more likely to trigger the development of pain or other somatic symptoms (44). Naturally occurring catastrophic events such as earthquakes, floods, or fires are much less likely to lead to chronic somatic symptoms than similarly stressful events that are "artificial" such as chemical spills or war (54). Being exposed to a multitude of stressors simultaneously, or over a period of time, may also be a significant risk for later somatic symptoms and/or psychological sequelae. Intensely stressful events can lead to permanent changes in the activity of both mouse and human stress response systems (49,55).

To complete this vicious circle, these changes in baseline function of the stress response (i.e., of the autonomic and neuroendocrine systems—see the next section) that may occur following a stressor earlier in life have been shown to predict which symptom-free individuals without chronic pain or other somatic symptoms are more likely to develop these somatic symptoms. This has been noted both in population-based studies and in experiments where healthy young adults are deprived of regular sleep or exercise (56,57).

This theoretical link between stress, changes in stress axis activity, and subsequent susceptibility to develop somatic symptoms or syndromes is also supported by studies showing that patients with FM and related conditions may be more likely than nonaffected individuals to have experienced physical or sexual abuse in childhood (58–61). Twin studies have recently supported a link between posttraumatic stress disorder (PTSD) and trauma, and CWP (62). Just as a lack of or cessation of exercise following trauma seems to be associated with a higher likelihood of developing pain or other somatic symptoms, a recent study of Israeli war veterans with PTSD showed that those who exercised regularly were much less likely to develop CWP or FM (63).

Role of Neuroendocrine Abnormalities

Because of this link between exposure to "stressors" and the subsequent development of FM, the human stress systems have been extensively studied in this condition. These studies have generally shown alterations of the hypothalamic-pituitary-adrenal (HPA) axis and the sympathetic nervous system in FM and related conditions (64–69). Although these studies often note either hypo- or hyperactivity of both the HPA axis and sympathetic nervous system in individuals with FM and related conditions, the precise abnormality varies from study to study. Moreover, these studies only find "abnormal" HPA or autonomic function is a very small percentage of patients, and there is tremendous overlap between patients and controls in any of these studies.

The inconsistency of these findings should not be surprising, since nearly all of these studies were cross-sectional studies that assumed that if HPA and/or autonomic dysfunction were found in FM, it must have *caused* the pain and other symptoms. Data now suggest the opposite. As noted above, there are better data suggesting that (especially HPA abnormalities) might represent a diathesis or be *due to* the pain or early life stress, rather than causing it. In fact in two recent studies examining HPA function in FM, McLean showed that salivary cortisol levels covaried with pain levels, and that CSF levels of CRH were more closely related to an individual's pain level or a history of early life trauma than whether they were a FM patient or control (70,71). Since most previous studies of HPA and autonomic function in FM failed to control pain levels, a previous history of trauma, and PTSD or other comorbid disorders that could affect HPA or autonomic dysfunction, it is not surprising for these inconsistencies to occur.

Heart rate variability at baseline and in response to tilt table testing has been evaluated in patients with FM as a surrogate measure of autonomic function. The consistent and reproducible finding of lower baseline heart rate variability in FM compared to controls (in three cross-sectional studies by two different groups) makes it a more useful measure than tilt table testing (68,69,72). An abnormal drop in blood pressure or excessive rate of syncope during tilt table testing has been noted in two of three cross-sectional studies completed by three different groups (73,74). One study noted no difference between normals and controls using univariate analysis (75). Moreover, recent findings also suggest that aberrations in heart rate variability may predispose to FM symptoms (56,57,76), possibly identifying patients at risk. Also, a recent study showed that heart rate variability was normalized following exercise therapy, suggesting that this finding might also be an epiphenomenon due in part to deconditioning (77).

It is likely that these neurobiological alterations are shared with other syndromes that are known to be associated with HPA and/or autonomic function such as depression or PTSD. A model of susceptibility and development of these disorders, which takes into account both genetics and personality as risk factors, is illustrated in Figure 3. This recognizes the critical importance of stressors in "re-setting stress response systems," as well as other factors including (*i*) the role of behavioral adaptations to these stressors such as cessation of routine exercise and (*ii*) whether an individual is in an environment characterized by control or support.

Augmented Pain and Sensory Processing as a Hallmark of FM and Related Syndromes

Once FM is established, by far the most consistently detected objective abnormalities involve pain and sensory processing systems. Since FM is defined in part by tenderness, considerable work has been performed exploring the potential reason for this phenomenon. The results of two decades of psychophysical pressure pain testing in FM have been very instructive.

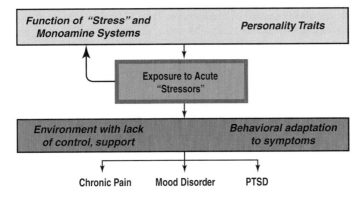

FIGURE 3 The hypothesized relationship between "stressors" and the development of syndromes such as fibromyalgia, PTSD, and depression.

One of the earliest findings in this regard was that the tenderness in FM is not confined to tender points, but instead extends throughout the entire body (29,31). Theoretically, such diffuse tenderness could be primarily due to either psychological (e.g., hypervigilance, where individuals are too attentive to their surroundings) or neurobiological (e.g., the plethora of factors that can lead to temporary or permanent amplification of sensory input) factors.

Early studies typically used dolorimetry to assess pressure pain threshold, and concluded that tenderness was in large part related to psychological factors, because these measures of pain threshold were correlated with levels of distress (31,32,78). Also, nuances such as the rate of increase of stimulus pressure, control by the operator versus control by the patient, and patient distress have been shown to influence pain threshold when it is measured in this manner (79,80).

To minimize the biases associated with "ascending" (i.e., the individual knows that the pressure will be predictably increased) measures of pressure pain threshold, Petzke and colleagues performed a series of studies using more sophisticated paradigms using random delivery of pressures (28,81,82). These studies showed that (*i*) the random measures of pressure pain threshold were not influenced by levels of distress of the individual, whereas tender point count and dolorimetry exams were; (*ii*) FM patients were much more sensitive to pressure even when these more sophisticated paradigms were used; (*iii*) FM patients were not any more "expectant" or "hypervigilant" than controls; and (*iv*) pressure pain thresholds at any four points in the body are highly correlated with the average tenderness at all 18 tender points and 4 control points (the thumbnail and forehead).

Because of this close link between tenderness and FM, this phenomenon has also been well studied as a potential relevant outcome in clinical trials of new FM therapies. In a number of longitudinal randomized placebo-controlled trials of FM, improvements in clinical pain have corresponded with a significant change in tender point counts or tender point index (83). In contrast, other studies did not show a correspondence between improvements in clinical pain and tender point counts (84–89). These discrepancies between previous studies could be either because these therapies did not improve tenderness or because tender points are not a good measure of tenderness. Two recent studies suggest the latter, because when individuals with FM were simultaneously assessed using tender point counts, dolorimetry, and random pressure paradigms, the random pressure paradigms showed the most responsiveness to change (90,91).

Heat, Cold, and Electrical Stimuli
In addition to the heightened sensitivity to pressure noted in FM, other types of stimuli applied to the skin are also judged as more painful or noxious by these patients. FM patients also display a decreased threshold to heat (82,92–94), cold (93,95), and electrical stimuli (96). Similar but somewhat attenuated decreases in pain threshold have also been noted in individuals with CWP without 11 or more tender points (97).

Responses to Other Sensory Stimuli
Gerster and colleagues were the first to demonstrate that FM patients also display a low noxious threshold to auditory tones, and this finding was subsequently replicated (98,99). However, both of these studies used ascending measures of auditory threshold, so these findings could theoretically be due to expectancy or hypervigilance. A recent study by Geisser and colleagues used identical random staircase paradigm to test FM patients' threshold to the loudness of auditory tones and to pressure (91). This study found that FM patients displayed low thresholds to both types of stimuli, and the correlation between the results of auditory and pressure pain threshold testing suggested that some of this was due to shared variance and some unique to one stimulus or the other. The notion that FM and related syndromes might represent biological amplification of all sensory stimuli has significant support from functional imaging studies that suggest that the insula is the most consistently hyperactive region (see below). This region has been noted to play a critical role in sensory integration, with the posterior insula serving a purer sensory role and the anterior insula being associated with the emotional processing of sensations (100–102).

Specific Mechanisms That May Lead to a Low Pain Threshold in FM
There are two different specific pathogenic mechanisms in FM that have been identified using experimental pain testing: (*i*) an absence of descending analgesic activity and (*ii*) increased wind-up or temporal summation.

Attenuated DNIC in FM. In healthy humans and laboratory animals, application of an intense painful stimulus for two to five minutes produces generalized whole-body analgesia. This analgesic effect, termed "diffuse noxious inhibitory controls" (DNIC), has been consistently observed to be attenuated or absent in groups of FM patients, compared to healthy controls (93,103–105). Wilder-Smith and colleagues have performed studies suggesting that in IBS there is a similar decrease in descending analgesic activity (106). A point of emphasis is that this finding of attenuated DNIC is not found in all FM or IBS patients, but is considerably more common in patients than controls.

The DNIC response in humans is believed to be partly mediated by descending opioidergic pathways and partly by descending serotonergic-noradrenergic pathways. In FM, the accumulating data suggest that opioidergic activity is normal or even increased, in that levels of cerebrospinal fluid (CSF) enkephalins are roughly twice as high in FM and idiopathic low back pain patients as in healthy controls (107). Moreover, positron emission tomography (PET) data show that baseline μ-opioid receptor binding is decreased in multiple pain processing regions in the brain of FM patients, consistent (but not pathognomonic) with the hypothesis that there is increased release of endogenous μ-opioid ligands in FM leading to high baseline occupancy of the receptors (108).

The biochemical and imaging findings suggesting increased activity of endogenous opioidergic systems in FM are consistent with the anecdotal experience that opioids are generally ineffective analgesics in patients with FM and related conditions. In contrast, studies have shown the opposite for serotonergic and noradrenergic activities in FM. Studies have shown that the principal metabolite of norepinephrine, 3-methoxy-4-hydroxyphenethylene (MPHG), is lower in the CSF of FM patients (109). Similarly, there are data suggesting low serotonin in this syndrome. Patients with FM were shown to have reduced serum levels of serotonin and its precursor, L-tryptophan, as well as reduced levels of the principal serotonin metabolite, 5-HIAA, in their CSF (109,110). Further evidence for this mechanism comes from treatment studies, where nearly any type of compound that simultaneously raises both serotonin and norepinephrine (tricyclics, duloxetine, milnacipran, tramadol) has been shown to be efficacious in treating FM and related conditions (89,111–113).

Increased wind-up in FM. Experimental pain testing studies have also suggested that some individuals with FM may have evidence of wind-up, indicative of evidence of central sensitization (114,115). In animal models, this finding is associated with excitatory amino acid and substance P hyperactivity (116–118). Just as with the findings regarding DNIC above, these results of psychophysical pain testing are congruent with both levels of neurotransmitters in the CSF, as well as clinical trials of drugs. Four independent studies have shown that patients with FM have approximately threefold higher concentrations of substance P in CSF when compared with normal controls (119–122) (Fig. 4). Other chronic pain syndromes, such as osteoarthritis (OA) of the hip and chronic low back pain, are also associated with elevated substance P levels, although chronic fatigue syndrome (which is not defined on the basis of pain) is not. Interestingly, once elevated, substance P levels do not appear to change dramatically and do not rise in response to acute painful stimuli. Thus, high substance P appears to be a biological marker for the presence of chronic pain.

Another important neurotransmitter in pain processing, and one that likely is playing some role in FM, is glutamate (Glu). It is a major excitatory neurotransmitter within the central nervous system; CSF levels of Glu are twice as high in FM patients than controls (123). Not only are these levels elevated, but a recent study using proton spectroscopy demonstrated that the Glu levels in the insula in FM change in response to changes in both clinical and experimental pain when patients are treated with acupuncture (124).

Nerve growth factor (NGF) and calcitonin gene-related peptide (CGRP) are additional neuropeptides that have been evaluated in FM. NGF was shown

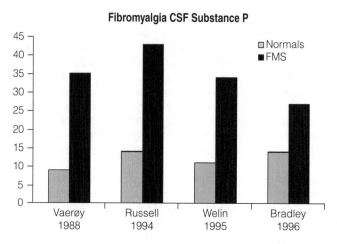

FIGURE 4 Levels of CSF levels of substance P in four different studies of FM.

Descending Influences on Nociceptive Processing

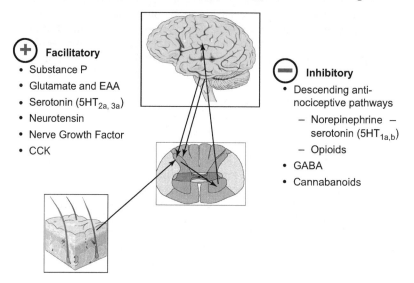

FIGURE 5 Neurotransmitters that are known to play either facilitatory (increase pain transmission) or inhibitory (decrease pain transmission) roles in the central nervous system.

in one study to have increased levels in FM, whereas CSF and serum CGRP have been studied and not found to be different in FM patients and controls (124–126).

Thus, a number of lines of evidence point to the fact that FM is a state of heightened pain or sensory processing, and that this might occur because of high levels of neurotransmitters that increase pain transmission and/or low levels of neurotransmitters that decrease pain transmission (Fig. 5).

Abnormalities on Functional Neuroimaging

Functional neural imaging enables investigators to visualize how the brain processes the sensory experience of pain. The primary modes of functional imaging that have been used in FM include functional magnetic resonance imaging (fMRI), single photon emission computed tomography (SPECT), PET, and proton spectroscopy (H-MRS).

Single-Photon Emission Computed Tomography (SPECT)

SPECT was the first functional neuroimaging technique to be used in FM. SPECT imaging involves the introduction of radioactive compounds into the participant's blood stream, which then decay over time giving a window for neural activity assessment. The first trial using SPECT imaging in FM patients was conducted by Mountz et al. (128). Their data from 10 FM patients and 7 age- and education-matched healthy controls indicated that both the caudate and the thalamus of FM patients had decreased blood flow. The findings by Mountz et al. were largely replicated in a second SPECT study by Kwiatek et al. (129). In a third SPECT trial, Guedj et al. reported a study using a more sensitive radi- oligand (99mTc-ECD) in FM patients and pain-free controls (130,131). Guedj et al. found hyperperfusion in FM patients within the somatosensory cortex and hypoperfusion in the anterior and posterior cingulate, the amygdala, medial frontal and parahippocampal gyrus, and the cerebellum. Finally, if these regional blood flow differences are relevant for FM pathology, one could hypothesize that changes in regional cerebral blood flow (rCBF) should track with changes in pain symptoms over time. One longitudinal treatment trial used SPECT imaging to assess changes in rCBF following administration of ami- triptyline within 14 FM patients (132). After three months of treatment with amitriptyline, increases in rCBF in the bilateral thalamus and the basal ganglia were observed. Since the same two regions had been implicated previously, these data suggest that amitriptyline may normalize the altered blood flow thereby reducing pain symptoms.

Functional MRI

fMRI is a noninvasive brain imaging technique that relies on changes in the relative concentration of oxygenated to deoxygenated hemoglobin within the brain. In response to neural activity, oxygenated blood flow is increased within the local brain area. This causes a decrease in the concentration of deoxygenated hemoglobin. Since deoxygenated hemoglobin is paramagnetic, this in turn causes a change in the magnetic property of the tissue. Unlike SPECT and PET, which can measure baseline levels of blood flow, the fMRI BOLD signal origi- nates from a difference between experimental conditions and does not assess baseline blood flow. Typically in FM trials involving fMRI, evoked pain sen- sations are compared to "off" conditions that have either no pain or involve an innocuous sensation.

The first study to use fMRI in FM patients was performed by Gracely et al. In this study, 16 FM patients and 16 matched controls were exposed to painful pressures during the fMRI experiment (133). The authors found increased neural activations (i.e., increase in the BOLD signal) in patients compared to pain-free controls when stimuli of equal pressure magnitude were administered. Regions of increased activity included the primary and secondary somatosensory cortex,

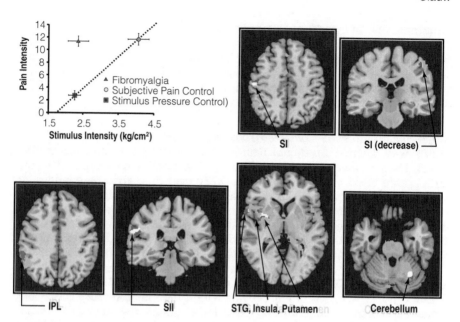

FIGURE 6 In top left panel, individuals with fibromyalgia (*triangle*) given a low-pressure stimulus have similar levels of pain, and of neuronal activation in areas of the brain known to be involved in pain processing (ends of *arrows*) as controls given nearly twice as much pressure. Controls given the same low pressure that causes pain in fibromyalgia rate their pain as 2/20 instead of 12/20 and have no neuronal activation with this amount of pressure.

the insula, and the anterior cingulate, all regions commonly observed in fMRI studies of healthy normal subjects during painful stimuli. Interestingly, when the pain-free controls were subjected to pressures that evoked equivalent pain ratings in the FM patients, similar activation patterns were observed. These findings were entirely consistent with the "left-shift" in stimulus-response function noted with experimental pain testing, and suggest that FM patients experience an increased gain or "volume setting" in brain sensory processing systems (Fig. 6). In a similar experiment, Cook et al. used painful heat stimuli during fMRI (134). Similar to the findings of Gracely et al., the authors observed significant increases in the pain ratings of patients and augmented pain processing within the contralateral insula. fMRI has also proved useful in determining how comorbid psychological factors influence pain processing in FM. For example, a recent study by Giesecke et al. explored the relationship between depression and enhanced evoked pain sensations in 30 patients with FM (135). The authors found that the anterior insula and amygdala activations were correlated with depressive symptoms, consistent with these regions being involved with affective or motivational aspects of pain processing. However, the degree of neuronal activation in areas of the brain thought to be associated with the "sensory" processing of pain (i.e., where the pain is localized and how intense it is) were not associated with levels of depressive symptoms, or the presence or absence of major depression. These data are consistent with a plethora of evidence in the pain field that there are different regions of the brain responsible for pain processing devoted to sensory intensity versus affective aspects of pain sensation, and suggest that the former and latter are largely independent of each other. In contrast, this same group showed that the presence of catastrophizing, a patient's negative or pessimistic appraisal of their pain, influences both the sensory and affective dimensions of pain on fMRI in FM (136).

Positron Emission Tomography
PET has been used in several studies in FM. In the first such study, Yunus and colleagues did not identify any differences in regional cerebral blood flow between FM patients and controls (137). However, Wood and colleagues used PET to show that attenuated dopaminergic activity may be playing a role in pain transmission in FM, and Harris and colleagues showed evidence of decreased μ-opiod receptor availability (possibly due to increased release of endogenous μ-opioids) in FM.

Other Biochemical and Cytokine Abnormalities
The amino acid tryptophan and the cytokine IL-8 have both been shown to be different in patients compared to controls in a couple of studies, but none have been evaluated in longitudinal studies (138–141). Low tryptophan, a precursor for serotonin, has been found in two of three studies by three different groups (138) (110,142). IL-8 has been consistently demonstrated in three studies by two different groups (139–141). Moreover, IL-8 has been shown to correlate with symptoms and not be associated with depressed FM. IL-8 levels are closely tied to autonomic function and these increased levels could be due to the dysautonomia seen in FM and related conditions (143). Serum IL-6 was evaluated and found to be normal in FM (141,144).

Structural Abnormalities in FM
Although a few studies have found mild abnormalities in the *skeletal muscles* of FM patients [these findings have been inconsistent and may be due to deconditioning rather than the illness itself (145–147)], there are a few studies that suggest there may be subsets of FM patients with damage to *neural* structures. P31-spectroscopy has been used to examine muscle metabolism in FM and the results are conflicting, with one study comparing sedentary controls to FM finding no differences and the other study finding lower ATP levels among FM patients (148,149). Studies suggest that the tenderness in FM is not at all confined to just the muscle, so in aggregate most investigators have concluded that primary muscle disease is not a likely cause of the pain associated with FM.

There are recent data, however, suggesting that a subset of FM patients may have abnormalities involving small sensory nerves in the skin, indicative of a small fiber neuropathy (150,151). There are also emerging data suggesting that there may be subtle abnormalities in brain structure seen in FM (152,153). Thus, if there are structural abnormalities or damage to tissues in FM, the most evidence for this is involving neural tissues.

Sleep in FM
In addition to pain, another symptom very commonly seen in FM is insomnia and disturbed sleep. One of the first biological findings in FM was that selective

sleep deprivation led to symptoms of FM in healthy individuals, and these findings have subsequently been replicated by several groups (18,154). However, the EEG abnormalities that were noted in this first study and initially thought to be a marker for FM, so-called α-intrusions, have subsequently been found to be present in normals and in individuals with other conditions (155,156). More recent findings on polysomnography that occur more commonly in FM include demonstration of fewer sleep spindles, an increase in cyclic alternating pattern rate, upper airway resistance syndrome, and/or poor sleep efficiency (157–160). However, sleep abnormalities rarely are shown to correlate with symptoms in FM, and many investigators anecdotally feel as though even identifying and treating specific sleep disorders often seen in FM patients (e.g., obstructive sleep apnea, upper airway resistance, restless leg or periodic limb movement syndromes) does not necessarily lead to improvements in the core symptoms of FM.

Behavioral and Psychological Factors

In addition to neurobiological mechanisms, behavioral and psychological factors also play a role in symptom expression in many FM patients. The rate of current psychiatric comorbidity in patients with FM may be as high as 30% to 60% in tertiary care settings, and the rate of lifetime psychiatric disorders even higher (3,161,162). Depression and anxiety disorders are the most commonly seen. However, these rates may be artifactually elevated by virtue of the fact that most of these studies have been performed in tertiary care centers. Individuals who meet ACR criteria for FM and who are identified in the general population do not have nearly this high a rate of identifiable psychiatric conditions (9,163) (Fig. 7).

As already noted, population-based studies have demonstrated that the relationship between pain and distress is complex and that distress is both a cause and consequence of pain. In this latter instance, a typical pattern is that as a result of pain and other symptoms of FM, individuals begin to function less well in their various roles. They may have difficulties with spouses, children, and work inside or outside the home, which exacerbate symptoms and lead to

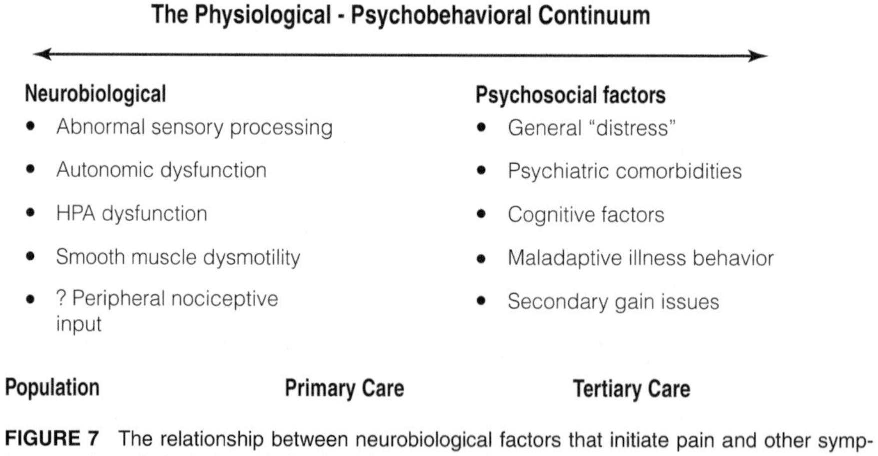

The Physiological - Psychobehavioral Continuum

←——→

Neurobiological
- Abnormal sensory processing
- Autonomic dysfunction
- HPA dysfunction
- Smooth muscle dysmotility
- ? Peripheral nociceptive input

Psychosocial factors
- General "distress"
- Psychiatric comorbidities
- Cognitive factors
- Maladaptive illness behavior
- Secondary gain issues

Population   **Primary Care**   **Tertiary Care**

FIGURE 7 The relationship between neurobiological factors that initiate pain and other symptoms, and psychological and behavioral factors that either preexist or develop as a result of pain and can perpetuate or worsen symptoms. These latter factors increase in frequency as one moves from examining pain in patients in the population to those seen in tertiary care centers.

maladaptive illness behaviors. These include isolation, cessation of pleasurable activities, reductions in activity and exercise, etc. In the worst cases, patients become involved with disability and compensation systems that almost ensure that they will not improve (164).

The complex interaction of biological, behavioral, psychological and cognitive mechanisms is not, however, unique to FM. Nonbiological factors play a prominent role in symptom expression in all rheumatic diseases. In fact, in conditions such as RA and OA, nonbiological factors such as level of formal education, coping strategies, and socioeconomic variables account for more of the variance in pain report and disability than biological factors such as the joint space width or sedimentation rate (165,166).

Because of the biopsychosocial nature of FM, several groups have attempted to identify subgroups of individuals with this condition, which may present differently or respond differentially to treatment (167,168). One of these studies examined how differential degrees of depression, maladaptive cognitions, and hyperalgesia might interact to lead to different subgroups of patients. Three identified subgroups can be usefully identified (Fig. 8). The first comprises approximately half of the patients who have low levels of depression and anxiety, normal cognition regarding pain, and are mildly tender (although tender enough to meet the ACR criteria). The second subgroup, representative of a "tertiary care" FM patient, is slightly more tender and also displays high levels of depression. These patients also have cognitions associated with a poor prognosis in many pain conditions. These include an external locus of pain control, defined as feeling that they can do nothing about their pain, and catastrophizing, defined as having a very negative and pessimistic view of their pain. The third subgroup, perhaps the most interesting, is the most tender but with no negative psychological or cognitive factors. This suggests that in some "resilient" individuals, positive psychological and cognitive factors issues may actually "buffer" neurobiological factors leading to pain and other symptoms in FM.

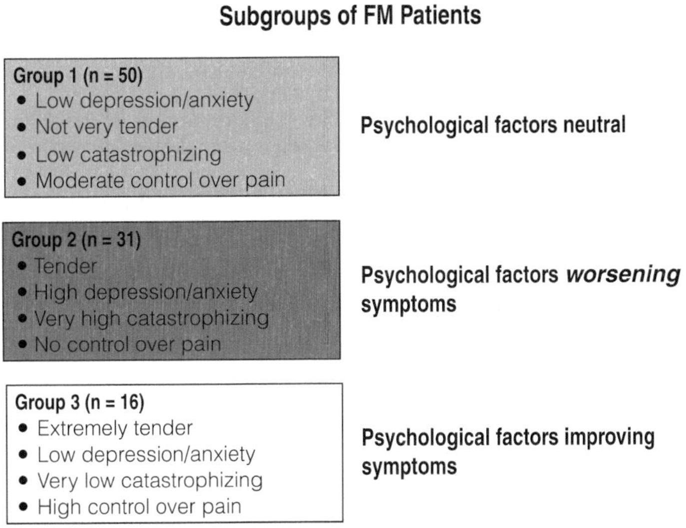

Subgroups of FM Patients

Group 1 (n = 50)
- Low depression/anxiety
- Not very tender
- Low catastrophizing
- Moderate control over pain

Psychological factors neutral

Group 2 (n = 31)
- Tender
- High depression/anxiety
- Very high catastrophizing
- No control over pain

Psychological factors *worsening* symptoms

Group 3 (n = 16)
- Extremely tender
- Low depression/anxiety
- Very low catastrophizing
- High control over pain

Psychological factors improving symptoms

FIGURE 8   Subgroups of fibromyalgia patients based on grouping by psychological, cognitive, and neurobiological (degree of hyperalgesia) factors.

Functional imaging studies have been instructive with regard to how these comorbid mood disorders or cognitions may be influencing pain processing in FM. The fMRI undertaken on 30 FM patients with variable levels of depression, with additional experimental pain testing, investigated how the presence or absence of depression influenced pain report (135). This study found that the level of depressive symptomatology did not influence the degree of neuronal activation in brain regions responsible for coding for the sensory intensity of pain, the primary and secondary somatosensory cortices. As expected, the depressed individuals did display greater activations in brain regions known to be responsible for the affective or cognitive processing of pain, such as the amygdala and insula. Another study with similar methodology examined how the presence or absence of catastrophizing might influence pain report in FM (136). In contrast to the results above, the presence of catastrophizing was associated with increased neuronal activations in the sensory coding regions. These studies thus provide empirical evidence for the value of treatments such as cognitive behavioral therapy. This is especially the case if individuals exhibit cognitions such as catastrophizing that, independent of other factors, may be capable of increasing pain intensity.

REFERENCES

1. Khan AA, Khan A, Harezlak J, et al. Somatic symptoms in primary care: etiology and outcome. Psychosomatics 2003; 44(6):471–478.
2. Mayer EA, Raybould HE. Role of visceral afferent mechanisms in functional bowel disorders. Gastroenterology 1990; 99(6):1688–1704.
3. Hudson JI, Hudson MS, Pliner LF, et al. Fibromyalgia and major affective disorder: a controlled phenomenology and family history study. Am J Psychiatry 1985; 142(4):441–446.
4. Arnold LM, Hudson JI, Hess EV, et al. Family study of fibromyalgia. Arthritis Rheum 2004; 50(3):944–952.
5. Wessely S, Nimnuan C, Sharpe M. Functional somatic syndromes: one or many? Lancet 1999; 354(9182):936–939.
6. Barsky AJ, Borus JF. Functional somatic syndromes. Ann Intern Med 1999; 130(11):910–921.
7. Fukuda K, Nisenbaum R, Stewart G, et al. Chronic multisymptom illness affecting Air Force veterans of the Gulf War. JAMA 1998; 280(11):981–988.
8. Drossman DA, Li ZM, Andruzzi E, et al. U.S. householder survey of functional gastrointestinal disorders. Prevalence, sociodemography, and health impact. Dig Dis Sci 1993; 38(9):1569–1580.
9. Aaron LA, Bradley LA, Alarcon GS, et al. Psychiatric diagnoses in patients with fibromyalgia are related to health care-seeking behavior rather than to illness [see comments]. Arthritis Rheum 1996; 39(3):436–445.
10. Maixner W, Fillingim R, Booker D, et al. Sensitivity of patients with painful temporomandibular disorders to experimentally evoked pain. Pain 1995; 63(3):341–351.
11. Naliboff BD, Derbyshire SW, Munakata J, et al. Cerebral activation in patients with irritable bowel syndrome and control subjects during rectosigmoid stimulation. Psychosom Med 2001; 63(3):365–375.
12. Giesecke T, Gracely RH, Grant MA, et al. Evidence of augmented central pain processing in idiopathic chronic low back pain. Arthritis Rheum 2004; 50(2):613–623.
13. Giesecke J, Reed BD, Haefner HK, et al. Quantitative sensory testing in vulvodynia patients and increased peripheral pressure pain sensitivity. Obstet Gynecol 2004; 104(1):126–133.
14. Moshiree B, Price DD, Robinson ME, et al. Thermal and visceral hypersensitivity in irritable bowel syndrome patients with and without fibromyalgia. Clin J Pain 2007; 23(4):323–330.

15. Clauw DJ. Fibromyalgia: update on mechanisms and management. J Clin Rheumatol 2007; 13(2):102–109.
16. Woolf CJ. Pain: moving from symptom control toward mechanism-specific pharmacologic management. Ann Intern Med 2004; 140(6):441–451.
17. Smythe HA, Moldofsky H. Two contributions to understanding of the "fibrositis" syndrome. Bull Rheum Dis 1977; 28(1):928–931.
18. Moldofsky H, Scarisbrick P, England R, et al. Musculosketal symptoms and non-REM sleep disturbance in patients with "fibrositis syndrome" and healthy subjects. Psychosom Med 1975; 37(4):341–351.
19. Yunus M, Masi AT, Calabro JJ, et al. Primary fibromyalgia (fibrositis): clinical study of 50 patients with matched normal controls. Semin Arthritis Rheum 1981; 11(1):151–171.
20. Wolfe F, Smythe HA, Yunus MB, et al. The American College of Rheumatology 1990 criteria for the classification of fibromyalgia. report of the multicenter criteria committee. Arthritis Rheum 1990; 33(2):160–172.
21. Yunus MB. Towards a model of pathophysiology of fibromyalgia: aberrant central pain mechanisms with peripheral modulation. J Rheumatol 1992; 19(6):846–850.
22. Clauw DJ, Chrousos GP. Chronic pain and fatigue syndromes: overlapping clinical and neuroendocrine features and potential pathogenic mechanisms. Neuroimmunomodulation 1997; 4(3):134–153.
23. Coster L, Kendall S, Gerdle B, et al. Chronic widespread musculoskeletal pain—a comparison of those who meet criteria for fibromyalgia and those who do not. Eur J Pain 2008; 12(5):600–610.
24. Jacobsen S, Bredkjaer SR. The prevalence of fibromyalgia and widespread chronic musculoskeletal pain in the general population. Scand J Rheumatol 1992; 21(5):261–263.
25. Raspe H. [Rheumatism epidemiology in Europe]. Soz Praventivmed 1992; 37(4):168–178.
26. Peleg R, Ablin JN, Peleg A, et al. Characteristics of fibromyalgia in Muslim Bedouin women in a primary care clinic. Semin Arthritis Rheum 2008; 37(6):398–402.
27. White KP, Thompson J. Fibromyalgia syndrome in an Amish community: a controlled study to determine disease and symptom prevalence. J Rheumatol 2003; 30(8):1835–1840.
28. Petzke F, Khine A, Williams D, et al. Dolorimetry performed at 3 paired tender points highly predicts overall tenderness. J Rheumatol 2001; 28(11):2568–2569.
29. Granges G, Littlejohn G. Pressure pain threshold in pain-free subjects, in patients with chronic regional pain syndromes, and in patients with fibromyalgia syndrome. Arthritis Rheum 1993; 36(5):642–646.
30. Cohen ML, Quintner J. Fibromyalgia syndrome, a problem of tautology. Lancet 1993; 342(8876):906–909.
31. Wolfe F, Ross K, Anderson J, et al. Aspects of fibromyalgia in the general population: sex, pain threshold, and fibromyalgia symptoms. J Rheumatol 1995; 22(1):151–156.
32. Wolfe F. The relation between tender points and fibromyalgia symptom variables: evidence that fibromyalgia is not a discrete disorder in the clinic. Ann Rheum Dis 1997; 56(4):268–271.
33. Buskila D, Neumann L, Hazanov I, et al. Familial aggregation in the fibromyalgia syndrome. Semin Arthritis Rheum 1996; 26(3):605–611.
34. Kato K, Sullivan PF, Evengard B, et al. Chronic widespread pain and its comorbidities: a population-based study. Arch Intern Med 2006; 166(15):1649–1654.
35. Hudson JI, Goldenberg DL, Pope HGJ, et al. Comorbidity of fibromyalgia with medical and psychiatric disorders. Am J Med 1993; 92(4):363–367.
36. Yunus MB. Central sensitivity syndromes: a new paradigm and group nosology for fibromyalgia and overlapping conditions, and the related issue of disease versus illness. Semin Arthritis Rheum 2008; 37(6):339–352.
37. Fukuda K, Dobbins JG, Wilson LJ, et al. An epidemiologic study of fatigue with relevance for the chronic fatigue syndrome. J Psychiatr Res 1997; 31(1):19–29.
38. Kato K, Sullivan PF, Evengard B, et al. Importance of genetic influences on chronic widespread pain. Arthritis Rheum 2006; 54(5):1682–1686.

39. Bondy B, Spaeth M, Offenbaecher M, et al. The T102C polymorphism of the 5-HT2A-receptor gene in fibromyalgia. Neurobiol Dis 1999; 6(5):433–439.
40. Offenbaecher M, Bondy B, de Jonge S, et al. Possible association of fibromyalgia with a polymorphism in the serotonin transporter gene regulatory region. Arthritis Rheum 1999; 42(11):2482–2488.
41. Buskila D, Cohen H, Neumann L, et al. An association between fibromyalgia and the dopamine D4 receptor exon III repeat polymorphism and relationship to novelty seeking personality traits. Mol Psychiatry 2004; 9(8):730–731.
42. Buskila D. Genetics of chronic pain states. Best Pract Res Clin Rheumatol 2007; 21(3):535–547.
43. Buskila D, Neumann L, Vaisberg G, et al. Increased rates of fibromyalgia following cervical spine injury. A controlled study of 161 cases of traumatic injury [see comments]. Arthritis Rheum 1997; 40(3):446–452.
44. McLean SA, Clauw DJ. Predicting chronic symptoms after an acute "stressor" – lessons learned from 3 medical conditions. Med Hypotheses 2004; 63(4):653–658.
45. Unwin C, Blatchley N, Coker W, et al. Health of UK servicemen who served in Persian Gulf War. Lancet 1999; 353(9148):169–178.
46. Hyams KC, Wignall FS, Roswell R. War syndromes and their evaluation: from the U.S. Civil War to the Persian Gulf War. Ann Intern Med 1996; 125(5):398–405.
47. Clauw DJ. The health consequences of the first Gulf War. BMJ 2003; 327:1357–1358.
48. Clauw DJ, Katz P. The overlap between fibromyalgia and inflammatory rheumatic diseases: when and why does it occur? J Clin Rheumatol 1995; 1:335–341.
49. Sapolsky RM. Why stress is bad for your brain. Science 1996; 273(5276):749–750.
50. Chrousos GP, Gold PW. The concepts of stress and stress system disorders. Overview of physical and behavioral homeostasis. JAMA 1992; 267(9):1244–1252.
51. Pillow DR, Zautra AJ, Sandler I. Major life events and minor stressors: identifying mediational links in the stress process. J Pers Soc Psychol 1996; 70(2):381–394.
52. Raphael KG, Natelson BH, Janal MN, et al. A community-based survey of fibromyalgia-like pain complaints following the World Trade Center terrorist attacks. Pain 2002; 100(1–2):131–139.
53. Williams DA, Brown SC, Clauw DJ, et al. Self-reported symptoms before and after September 11 in patients with fibromyalgia. JAMA 2003; 289(13):1637–1638.
54. Clauw DJ, Engel CC Jr, Aronowitz R, et al. Unexplained symptoms after terrorism and war: an expert consensus statement. J Occup Environ Med 2003; 45(10): 1040–1048.
55. Heim C, Newport DJ, Bonsall R, et al. Altered pituitary-adrenal axis responses to provocative challenge tests in adult survivors of childhood abuse. Am J Psychiatry 2001; 158(4):575–581.
56. Glass JM, Lyden A, Petzke F, et al. The effect of brief exercise cessation on pain, fatigue, and mood symptom development in healthy, fit individuals. J Psychosom Res 2004; 57(4):391–398.
57. McBeth J, Silman AJ, Gupta A, et al. Moderation of psychosocial risk factors through dysfunction of the hypothalamic-pituitary-adrenal stress axis in the onset of chronic widespread musculoskeletal pain: findings of a population-based prospective cohort study. Arthritis Rheum 2007; 56(1):360–371.
58. Aaron LA, Bradley LA, Alarcon GS, et al. Perceived physical and emotional trauma as precipitating events in fibromyalgia. Associations with health care seeking and disability status but not pain severity [see comments]. Arthritis Rheum 1997; 40(3): 453–460.
59. Alexander RW, Bradley LA, Alarcon GS, et al. Sexual and physical abuse in women with fibromyalgia: association with outpatient health care utilization and pain medication usage. Arthritis Care Res 1998; 11(2):102–115.
60. Boisset-Pioro MH, Esdaile JM, Fitzcharles MA. Sexual and physical abuse in women with fibromyalgia syndrome. Arthritis Rheum 1995; 38(2):235–241.
61. Drossman DA. Sexual and physical abuse and gastrointestinal illness. Scand J Gastroenterol Suppl 1995; 208:90–96.

62. Arguelles LM, Afari N, Buchwald DS, et al. A twin study of posttraumatic stress disorder symptoms and chronic widespread pain. Pain 2006; 124(1–2):150–157.
63. Arnson Y, Amital D, Fostick L, et al. Physical activity protects male patients with post-traumatic stress disorder from developing severe fibromyalgia. Clin Exp Rheumatol 2007; 25(4):529–533.
64. Crofford LJ, Pillemer SR, Kalogeras KT, et al. Hypothalamic-pituitary-adrenal axis perturbations in patients with fibromyalgia. Arthritis Rheum 1994; 37(11):1583–1592.
65. Demitrack MA, Crofford LJ. Evidence for and pathophysiologic implications of hypothalamic-pituitary-adrenal axis dysregulation in fibromyalgia and chronic fatigue syndrome. Ann N Y Acad Sci 1998; 840:684–697.
66. Qiao ZG, Vaeroy H, Morkrid L. Electrodermal and microcirculatory activity in patients with fibromyalgia during baseline, acoustic stimulation and cold pressor tests. J Rheumatol 1991; 18(9):1383–1389.
67. Adler GK, Kinsley BT, Hurwitz S, et al. Reduced hypothalamic-pituitary and sympathoadrenal responses to hypoglycemia in women with fibromyalgia syndrome. Am J Med 1999; 106(5):534–543.
68. Martinez-Lavin M, Hermosillo AG, Rosas M, et al. Circadian studies of autonomic nervous balance in patients with fibromyalgia: a heart rate variability analysis. Arthritis Rheum 1998; 41(11):1966–1971.
69. Cohen H, Neumann L, Shore M, et al. Autonomic dysfunction in patients with fibromyalgia: application of power spectral analysis of heart rate variability [see comments]. Semin Arthritis Rheum 2000; 29(4):217–227.
70. McLean SA, Williams DA, Harris RE, et al. Momentary relationship between cortisol secretion and symptoms in patients with fibromyalgia. Arthritis Rheum 2005; 52(11): 3660–3669.
71. McLean SA, Williams DA, Stein PK, et al. Cerebrospinal fluid corticotropin-releasing factor concentration is associated with pain but not fatigue symptoms in patients with fibromyalgia. Neuropsychopharmacology 2006; 31(12):2776–2782.
72. Cohen H, Buskila D, Neumann L, et al. Confirmation of an association between fibromyalgia and serotonin transporter promoter region (5-HTTLPR) polymorphism, and relationship to anxiety-related personality traits. Arthritis Rheum 2002; 46(3):845–847.
73. Bou-Holaigah I, Calkins H, Flynn JA, et al. Provocation of hypotension and pain during upright tilt table testing in adults with fibromyalgia. Clin Exp Rheumatol 1997; 15(3):239–246.
74. Naschitz JE, Rosner I, Rozenbaum M, et al. The capnography head-up tilt test for evaluation of chronic fatigue syndrome. Semin Arthritis Rheum 2000; 30(2):79–86.
75. Rosner I, Rozenbaum M, Naschitz JE, et al. Cardiovascular response to upright tilt differs in fibromyalgia from chronic fatigue syndrome. American College of Rheumatology [Poster Session C Fibromyalgia and Soft Tissue Rheumatism I], 2000; S209.
76. McBeth J, Jones K. Epidemiology of chronic musculoskeletal pain. Best Pract Res Clin Rheumatol 2007; 21(3):403–425.
77. Figueroa A, Kingsley JD, McMillan V, et al. Resistance exercise training improves heart rate variability in women with fibromyalgia. Clin Physiol Funct Imaging 2008; 28(1):49–54.
78. Gracely RH, Grant MA, Giesecke T. Evoked pain measures in fibromyalgia. Best Pract Res Clin Rheumatol 2003; 17(4):593–609.
79. Jensen K, Andersen HO, Olesen J, et al. Pressure-pain threshold in human temporal region. Evaluation of a new pressure algometer. Pain 1986; 25(3):313–323.
80. Petzke F, Gracely RH, Park KM, et al. What do tender points measure? Influence of distress on 4 measures of tenderness. J Rheumatol 2003; 30(3):567–574.
81. Petzke F, Gracely RH, Khine A, et al. Pain sensitivity in patients with fibromyalgia (FM): expectancy effects on pain measurements. Arthritis Rheum 1999; 42(suppl 9): S342.
82. Petzke F, Clauw DJ, Ambrose K, et al. Increased pain sensitivity in fibromyalgia: effects of stimulus type and mode of presentation. Pain 2003; 105(3):403–413.

83. Farber L, Stratz T, Bruckle W, et al. Efficacy and tolerability of tropisetron in primary fibromyalgia—A highly selective and competitive 5-HT3 receptor antagonist. German Fibromyalgia Study Group. Scand J Rheumatol Suppl 2000; 113:49–54.
84. Arnold LM, Hess EV, Hudson JI, et al. A randomized, placebo-controlled, double-blind, flexible-dose study of fluoxetine in the treatment of women with fibromyalgia. Am J Med 2002; 112(3):191–197.
85. Goldenberg D, Mayskiy M, Mossey C, et al. A randomized, double-blind crossover trial of fluoxetine and amitriptyline in the treatment of fibromyalgia. Arthritis Rheum 1996; 39(11):1852–1859.
86. Gowans SE, de Hueck A, Voss S, et al. Effect of a randomized, controlled trial of exercise on mood and physical function in individuals with fibromyalgia. Arthritis Rheum 2001; 45(6):519–529.
87. Jacobsen S, Danneskiold-Samsoe B, Andersen RB. Oral S-adenosylmethionine in primary fibromyalgia. Double-blind clinical evaluation. Scand J Rheumatol 1991; 20(4):294–302.
88. Scudds RA, McCain GA, Rollman GB, et al. Improvements in pain responsiveness in patients with fibrositis after successful treatment with amitriptyline. J Rheumatol Suppl 1989; 19:98–103.
89. Arnold LM, Keck PEJ, Welge JA. Antidepressant treatment of fibromyalgia. A meta-analysis and review. Psychosomatics 2000; 41(2):104–113.
90. Harris RE, Gracely RH, McLean SA, et al. Comparison of clinical and evoked pain measures in fibromyalgia. J Pain 2006; 7(7):521–527.
91. Geisser ME, Gracely RH, Giesecke T, et al. The association between experimental and clinical pain measures among persons with fibromyalgia and chronic fatigue syndrome. Eur J Pain 2007; 11(2):202–207.
92. Gibson SJ, Littlejohn GO, Gorman MM, et al. Altered heat pain thresholds and cerebral event-related potentials following painful CO_2 laser stimulation in subjects with fibromyalgia syndrome. Pain 1994; 58(2):185–193.
93. Kosek E, Hansson P. Modulatory influence on somatosensory perception from vibration and heterotopic noxious conditioning stimulation (HNCS) in fibromyalgia patients and healthy subjects. Pain 1997; 70(1):41–51.
94. Geisser ME, Casey KL, Brucksch CB, et al. Perception of noxious and innocuous heat stimulation among healthy women and women with fibromyalgia: association with mood, somatic focus, and catastrophizing. Pain 2003; 102(3):243–250.
95. Kosek E, Ekholm J, Hansson P. Sensory dysfunction in fibromyalgia patients with implications for pathogenic mechanisms. Pain 1996; 68(2–3):375–383.
96. Arroyo JF, Cohen ML. Abnormal responses to electrocutaneous stimulation in fibromyalgia. J Rheumatol 1993; 20(11):1925–1931.
97. Carli G, Suman AL, Biasi G, et al. Reactivity to superficial and deep stimuli in patients with chronic musculoskeletal pain. Pain 2002; 100(3):259–269.
98. Gerster JC, Hadj-Djilani A. Hearing and vestibular abnormalities in primary fibrositis syndrome. J Rheumatol 1984; 11(5):678–680.
99. McDermid AJ, Rollman GB, McCain GA. Generalized hypervigilance in fibromyalgia: evidence of perceptual amplification. Pain 1996; 66(2–3):133–144.
100. Tracey I, Mantyh PW. The cerebral signature for pain perception and its modulation. Neuron 2007; 55(3):377–391.
101. Craig AD. Human feelings: why are some more aware than others? Trends Cogn Sci 2004; 8(6):239–241.
102. Craig AD. Interoception: the sense of the physiological condition of the body. Curr Opin Neurobiol 2003; 13(4):500–505.
103. Lautenbacher S, Rollman GB. Possible deficiencies of pain modulation in fibromyalgia. Clin J Pain 1997; 13(3):189–196.
104. Leffler AS, Hansson P, Kosek E. Somatosensory perception in a remote pain-free area and function of diffuse noxious inhibitory controls (DNIC) in patients suffering from long-term trapezius myalgia. Eur J Pain 2002; 6(2):149–159.
105. Julien N, Goffaux P, Arsenault P, et al. Widespread pain in fibromyalgia is related to a deficit of endogenous pain inhibition. Pain 2005; 114(1–2):295–302.

106. Wilder-Smith CH, Robert-Yap J. Abnormal endogenous pain modulation and somatic and visceral hypersensitivity in female patients with irritable bowel syndrome. World J Gastroenterol 2007; 13(27):3699–3704.
107. Baraniuk JN, Whalen G, Cunningham J, et al. Cerebrospinal fluid levels of opioid peptides in fibromyalgia and chronic low back pain. BMC Musculoskelet Disord 2004; 5(1):48.
108. Harris RE, Clauw DJ, Scott DJ, et al. Decreased central mu-opioid receptor availability in fibromyalgia. J Neurosci 2007; 27(37):10000–10006.
109. Russell IJ, Vaeroy H, Javors M, et al. Cerebrospinal fluid biogenic amine metabolites in fibromyalgia/fibrositis syndrome and rheumatoid arthritis. Arthritis Rheum 1992; 35(5):550–556.
110. Yunus MB, Dailey JW, Aldag JC, et al. Plasma tryptophan and other amino acids in primary fibromyalgia: a controlled study. J Rheumatol 1992; 19(1):90–94.
111. Arnold LM, Lu Y, Crofford LJ, et al. A double-blind, multicenter trial comparing duloxetine with placebo in the treatment of fibromyalgia patients with or without major depressive disorder. Arthritis Rheum 2004; 50(9):2974–2984.
112. Bennett RM, Kamin M, Karim R, et al. Tramadol and acetaminophen combination tablets in the treatment of fibromyalgia pain: a double-blind, randomized, placebo-controlled study. Am J Med 2003; 114(7):537–545.
113. Gendreau RM, Thorn MD, Gendreau JF, et al. The efficacy of milnacipran in fibromyalgia. J Rheumatol 2005; 32(10):1975–1985.
114. Staud R, Vierck CJ, Cannon RL, et al. Abnormal sensitization and temporal summation of second pain (wind-up) in patients with fibromyalgia syndrome. Pain 2001; 91(1–2):165–175.
115. Price DD, Staud R, Robinson ME, et al. Enhanced temporal summation of second pain and its central modulation in fibromyalgia patients. Pain 2002; 99(1–2):49–59.
116. Woolf CJ, Thompson SW. The induction and maintenance of central sensitization is dependent on N-methyl-D-aspartic acid receptor activation; implications for the treatment of post-injury pain hypersensitivity states. Pain 1991; 44(3):293–299.
117. Woolf CJ. Windup and central sensitization are not equivalent. Pain 1996; 66(2–3): 105–108.
118. Xu XJ, Dalsgaard CJ, Wiesenfeld-Hallin Z. Spinal substance P and N-methyl-D-aspartate receptors are coactivated in the induction of central sensitization of the nociceptive flexor reflex. Neuroscience 1992; 51(3):641–648.
119. Welin M, Bragee B, Nyberg F, et al. Elevated substance P levels are contrasted by a decrease in met-enkephalin-arg-phe levels in CSF from fibromyalgia patients. J Muscoskel Pain 1995; 3(1):4.
120. Vaeroy H, Helle R, Forre O, et al. Elevated CSF levels of substance P and high incidence of Raynaud phenomenon in patients with fibromyalgia: new features for diagnosis. Pain 1988; 32(1):21–26.
121. Russell IJ, Orr MD, Littman B, et al. Elevated cerebrospinal fluid levels of substance P in patients with the fibromyalgia syndrome. Arthritis Rheum 1994; 37(11): 1593–1601.
122. Bradley LA, Alberts KR, Alarcon GS, et al. Abnormal brain regional cerebral blood flow and cerebrospinal fluid levels of Substance P in patients and non-patients with fibromyalgia. Arthritis Rheum 1996; 39(suppl 9):212 (abstr 1109).
123. Sarchielli P, Di Filippo M, Nardi K, et al. Sensitization, glutamate, and the link between migraine and fibromyalgia. Curr Pain Headache Rep 2007; 11(5):343–351.
124. Harris RE, Clauw DJ. How do we know that the pain in fibromyalgia is "real"? Curr Pain Headache Rep 2006; 10(6):403–407.
125. Giovengo SL, Russell IJ, Larson AA. Increased concentrations of nerve growth factor in cerebrospinal fluid of patients with fibromyalgia. J Rheumatol 1999; 26(7): 1564–1569.
126. Vaeroy H, Sakurada T, Forre O, et al. Modulation of pain in fibromyalgia (fibrositis syndrome): cerebrospinal fluid (CSF) investigation of pain related neuropeptides with special reference to calcitonin gene related peptide (CGRP). J Rheumatol Suppl 1989; 19:94–97.

127. Hocherl K, Farber L, Ladenburger S, et al. Effect of tropisetron on circulating cat-echolamines and other putative biochemical markers in serum of patients with fibromyalgia. Scand J Rheumatol Suppl 2000; 113:46–48.
128. Mountz JM, Bradley LA, Modell JG, et al. Fibromyalgia in women. Abnormalities of regional cerebral blood flow in the thalamus and the caudate nucleus are associated with low pain threshold levels. Arthritis Rheum 1995; 38(7):926–938.
129. Kwiatek R, Barnden L, Tedman R, et al. Regional cerebral blood flow in fibro-myalgia: single-photon-emission computed tomography evidence of reduction in the pontine tegmentum and thalami. Arthritis Rheum 2000; 43(12):2823–2833.
130. Guedj E, Taieb D, Cammilleri S, et al. 99mTc-ECD brain perfusion SPECT in hyperalgesic fibromyalgia. Eur J Nucl Med Mol Imaging 2007; 34(1):130–134.
131. Guedj E, Cammilleri S, Colavolpe C, et al. Predictive value of brain perfusion SPECT for ketamine response in hyperalgesic fibromyalgia. Eur J Nucl Med Mol Imaging 2007; 34(8):1274–1279.
132. Adiguzel O, Kaptanoglu E, Turgut B, et al. The possible effect of clinical recovery on regional cerebral blood flow deficits in fibromyalgia: a prospective study with semiquantitative SPECT. South Med J 2004; 97(7):651–655.
133. Gracely RH, Petzke F, Wolf JM, et al. Functional magnetic resonance imaging evidence of augmented pain processing in fibromyalgia. Arthritis Rheum 2002; 46(5):1333–1343.
134. Cook DB, Lange G, Ciccone DS, et al. Functional imaging of pain in patients with primary fibromyalgia. J Rheumatol 2004; 31(2):364–378.
135. Giesecke T, Gracely R H, Williams DA, et al. The relationship between depression, clinical pain, and experimental pain in a chronic pain cohort. Arthritis Rheum 2005; 52(5):1577–1584.
136. Gracely RH, Geisser ME, Giesecke T, et al. Pain catastrophizing and neural responses to pain among persons with fibromyalgia. Brain 2004; 127(pt 4):835–843.
137. Yunus MB, Young CS, Saeed AS, et al. Positron emission tomography (PET) imaging of the brain in fibromyalgia syndrome (FMS). Arthritis Rheum 1997; 40(95):S188.
138. Russell IJ, Michalek JE, Vipraio GA, et al. Serum amino acids in fibrositis/fibro-myalgia syndrome. J Rheumatol 1989; 19:158–163.
139. Wallace D, Bowman RL, Wormsley SB, et al. Cytokines and immune regulation in patients with fibrositis [letter]. Arthritis Rheum 1989; 32(10):1334–1335.Erratum in: Arthritis Rheum 1989; 32(12):1607.
140. Gur A, Karakoc M, Erdogan S, et al. Regional cerebral blood flow and cytokines in young females with fibromyalgia. Clin Exp Rheumatol 2002; 20(6):753–760.
141. Gur A, Karakoc M, Nas K, et al. Cytokines and depression in cases with fibro-myalgia. J Rheumatol 2002; 29(2):358–361.
142. Larson AA, Giovengo SL, Russell IJ, et al. Changes in the concentrations of amino acids in the cerebrospinal fluid that correlate with pain in patients with fibro-myalgia: implications for nitric oxide pathways. Pain 2000; 87(2):201–211.
143. Elenkov IJ, Wilder RL, Chrousos GP, et al. The sympathetic nerve–an integrative interface between two supersystems: the brain and the immune system. Pharmacol Rev 2000; 52(4):595–638.
144. Wallace DJ, Linker-Israeli M, Hallegua D, et al. Cytokines play an aetiopathogenetic role in fibromyalgia: a hypothesis and pilot study. Rheumatology (Oxford) 2001; 40 (7):743–749.
145. Drewes AM, Andreasen A, Schroder HD, et al. Pathology of skeletal muscle in fibromyalgia: a histo-immuno-chemical and ultrastructural study. Br J Rheumatol 1993; 32(6):479–483.
146. Bennett RM, Jacobsen S. Muscle function and origin of pain in fibromyalgia. Bail-lieres Clin Rheumatol 1994; 8(4):721–746.
147. Geel SE. The fibromyalgia syndrome: musculoskeletal pathophysiology. Semin Arthritis Rheum 1994; 23(5):347–353.
148. Simms RW, Roy SH, Hrovat M, et al. Lack of association between fibromyalgia syndrome and abnormalities in muscle energy metabolism. Arthritis Rheum 1994; 37(6):794–800.

149. Park JH, Phothimat P, Oates CT, et al. Use of P-31 magnetic resonance spectroscopy to detect metabolic abnormalities in muscles of patients with fibromyalgia. Arthritis Rheum 1998; 41(3):406–413.

150. Caro XJ, Winter EF, Dumas AJ. A subset of fibromyalgia patients have findings suggestive of chronic inflammatory demyelinating polyneuropathy and appear to respond to IVIg. Rheumatology (Oxford) 2008; 47(2):208–211.

151. Kim SH, Kim DH, Oh DH, et al. Characteristic electron microscopic findings in the skin of patients with fibromyalgia-preliminary study. Clin Rheumatol 2008; 27(3):407–411.

152. Sundgren PC, Petrou M, Harris RE, et al. Diffusion-weighted and diffusion tensor imaging in fibromyalgia patients: a prospective study of whole brain diffusivity, apparent diffusion coefficient, and fraction anisotropy in different regions of the brain and correlation with symptom severity. Acad Radiol 2007; 14(7):839–846.

153. Kuchinad A, Schweinhardt P, Seminowicz DA, et al. Accelerated brain gray matter loss in fibromyalgia patients: premature aging of the brain? J Neurosci 2007; 27(15):4004–4007.

154. Older SA, Battafarano DF, Danning CL, et al. The effects of delta wave sleep interruption on pain thresholds and fibromyalgia-like symptoms in healthy subjects; correlations with insulin-like growth factor I. J Rheumatol 1998; 25(6):1180–1186.

155. Branco J, Atalaia A, Paiva T. Sleep cycles and alpha-delta sleep in fibromyalgia syndrome. J Rheumatol 1994; 21(6):1113–1117.

156. Drewes AM, Svendsen L. Quantification of alpha-EEG activity during sleep in fibromyalgia: a study based on ambulatory sleep monitoring. J Musculoskel Pain 1994; 2(4):33–53.

157. Landis CA, Lentz MJ, Rothermel J, et al. Decreased sleep spindles and spindle activity in midlife women with fibromyalgia and pain. Sleep 2004; 27(4):741–750.

158. Rizzi M, Sarzi-Puttini P, Atzeni F, et al. Cyclic alternating pattern: a new marker of sleep alteration in patients with fibromyalgia? J Rheumatol 2004; 31(6):1193–1199.

159. Sarzi-Puttini P, Rizzi M, Andreoli A, et al. Hypersomnolence in fibromyalgia syndrome. Clin Exp Rheumatol 2002; 20(1):69–72.

160. Sergi M, Rizzi M, Braghiroli A, et al. Periodic breathing during sleep in patients affected by fibromyalgia syndrome. Eur Respir J 1999; 14(1):203–208.

161. Boissevain MD, McCain GA. Toward an integrated understanding of fibromyalgia syndrome. I. Medical and pathophysiological aspects. Pain 1991; 45(3):227–238.

162. Epstein SA, Kay GG, Clauw DJ, et al. Psychiatric disorders in patients with fibromyalgia. A multicenter investigation. Psychosomatics 1999; 40(1):57–63.

163. White KP, Nielson WR, Harth M, et al. Does the label "fibromyalgia" alter health status, function, and health service utilization? A prospective, within-group comparison in a community cohort of adults with chronic widespread pain. Arthritis Rheum 2002; 47(3):260–265.

164. Hadler NM. If you have to prove you are ill, you can't get well. The object lesson of fibromyalgia. Spine 1996; 21(20):2397–2400.

165. Hawley DJ, Wolfe F. Pain, disability, and pain/disability relationships in seven rheumatic disorders: a study of 1,522 patients. J Rheumatol 1991; 18(10):1552–1557.

166. Callahan LF, Smith WJ, Pincus T. Self-report questionnaires in five rheumatic diseases: comparisons of health status constructs and associations with formal education level. Arthritis Care Res 1989; 2(4):122–131.

167. Turk DC, Okifuji A, Sinclair JD, et al. Pain, disability, and physical functioning in subgroups of patients with fibromyalgia. J Rheumatol 1996; 23(7):1255–1262.

168. Giesecke T, Williams DA, Harris RE, et al. Subgrouping of fibromyalgia patients on the basis of pressure-pain thresholds and psychological factors. Arthritis Rheum 2003; 48(10):2916–2922.

2

Evaluation

Leslie J. Crofford
Division of Rheumatology and Women's Health, and Center for the Advancement of Women's Health, University of Kentucky, Lexington, Kentucky, U.S.A.

INTRODUCTION

The typical chief complaint of a patient who is ultimately diagnosed with fibromyalgia (FM) is "I hurt all over." However, musculoskeletal pain, even widespread pain, is a very common complaint in the primary care setting, and assuring that patients who present with symptoms of widespread pain have FM and do not have other causes for their symptoms can be a daunting task. Further complicating the evaluation, FM is often comorbid with other conditions and optimum management will require addressing both conditions. It is imperative for physicians to separate for themselves, and for their patients, what complaints should properly be attributed to FM and what symptoms should be attributed to other conditions. This can be challenging but is crucial for creating a framework by which treatment effects can be evaluated and for educating patients about the intended outcomes of treatment or combination of treatments.

PRESENTING SYMPTOMS

Pain

The pain of FM involves muscles, joints, and even skin. It must be present above and below the waist on both sides of the body and involve the axial skeleton (neck, back, or chest) (1). Shoulder and buttock pain, if bilateral, is considered as both sides of the body. The pain attributable to FM is poorly localized, difficult to ignore, severe in its characterization, and associated with reduction in the capacity to fulfill roles and responsibilities (2). Musculoskeletal pain must be chronic to make the diagnosis of FM, and chronic means that the pain is present most of the day on most days for at least three months.

In taking the history of patients with widespread pain, it is useful to pay attention to particular body areas that are more severely affected. This can be done by asking the patient to identify the top three painful areas, or by using a body map and having the patient shade areas dark or light according to the intensity of the pain (Fig. 1). The purpose is to identify potential pain generators that may not be attributable to FM per se, and therefore responsive to specific treatments. For example, a patient may have a specific complaint associated with bursitis, tendonitis, or arthritis that would respond to local injection (e.g., rotator cuff, trochanteric bursitis, osteoarthritis of the knee) or anti-inflammatory/analgesic medications (e.g., nonsteroidal anti-inflammatory drugs or acetaminophen), which are not typically effective for the more widespread pain of FM.

Non-pain Symptoms

In addition to the required symptom of chronic widespread musculoskeletal pain, typical patients will complain of stiffness, fatigue, sleep disturbance, cognitive dysfunction, anxiety, and depression (3). These "fellow travelers" with pain are certainly not unique to FM, but can rise to a level that they are as

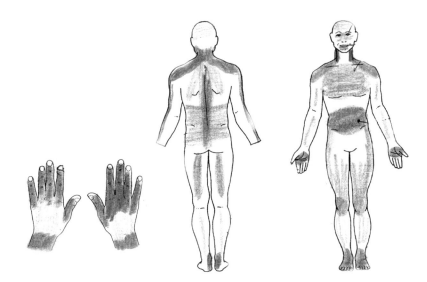

FIGURE 1 Pain body map.

distressing as pain and be of equal impact on function and quality of life. Although present to varying degrees in most patients with FM, these symptoms are not present in everyone or at all times.

Fatigue in particular is highly prevalent in primary care patients ultimately diagnosed with FM (4). Pain, stiffness, and fatigue are often worsened by physical activity (post-exertional malaise). Sleep complaints in FM can include difficulty falling asleep, staying asleep, or early awakening. Regardless of the specific complaint, patients awake feeling unrefreshed. The cognitive complaints are often characterized as slowness in cognitive processing, concentration problems, difficulties with word retrieval, and short-term memory problems (5,6). Most patients with any kind of illness associated with chronic pain and fatigue will have symptoms of anxiety and depression to a greater degree than healthy individuals. In patients with FM, anxiety may be even more common than depression (2,7). Patients should be screened for major depressive disorder by query for depressed mood (feeling down, depressed, or hopeless) and anhedonia (little interest or pleasure in activities).

Overlapping Syndromes

Because FM can overlap in presentation with other chronic pain conditions, the review of systems often includes headaches, facial/jaw pain, and other regional myofascial pain complaints particularly involving the neck and back pain (8–10). Furthermore, visceral pain complaints are often present involving gastrointestinal (GI), genitourinary (GU), and reproductive organs. GI complaints can include symptoms of gastroesophageal reflux and irritable bowel syndrome, including bloating, cramping, and alternating diarrhea and constipation (11). Irritable bladder/interstitial cystitis, painful bladder, or overactive bladder are often present and characterized by a combination of pelvic and/or perineal pain, frequent voiding day and night, urgency to urinate, and pain with holding urine (12).

The above associations are well supported in the literature, but patients with FM may also complain of symptoms not part of any defined clinical syndrome. Some of these can be characterized as neurosensory, such as a feeling of burning, numbness, tingling, or swelling in the extremities (3). Other sensory complaints include tinnitus or hyperacusis, vertigo, and visual changes or photophobia. Patients may complain of thermal instability.

Taking all the symptoms in aggregate, one may take the view that patients with FM are hyperaware of bodily sensations and perceive that the symptoms they experience may be threatening as has been shown in patients with visceral pain syndromes (13,14). When one takes into account that symptoms of FM often have their onset and are exacerbated during periods of high perceived stress, severity of FM symptoms may reflect an interaction between neurobiological pathways controlling somatic perception and central stress physiology, which is known to increase vigilance and enhance sensory processing (15).

Psychosocial History
Understanding current psychosocial stressors surrounding a patient's roles and responsibilities will aid the astute clinician in managing the patient with FM. Many factors that can exacerbate symptoms are not amenable to pharmacologic intervention, and having the patient recognize the impact of psychosocial factors on their symptoms can allay anxiety. Furthermore, the prevalence of exposure to major traumatic events, including interpersonal and other forms of violence, must be assessed (16). If posttraumatic stress disorder is an issue, the clinician should be aware and consider how treatment might be optimized.

DIFFERENTIAL DIAGNOSIS
Before completing the physical examination and determining which laboratory or radiographic tests are needed to evaluate the patient, it is useful to consider the differential diagnosis and ask additional questions that may help to guide the evaluation. Table 1 lists some of the more common conditions that should be considered.

Autoimmune Inflammatory Disorders
Because pain and fatigue are common complaints for patients with systemic inflammatory diseases, one should initially determine if the patient has an autoimmune inflammatory etiology or not. Patients with more than 6 to 12 months of symptoms typically have a relatively easily identifiable autoimmune inflammatory disorder if it is present. If the patient under consideration is more than 50 years, then polymyalgia rheumatica (PMR) should be considered. Symptoms of PMR include pain and stiffness, localized primarily to the shoulder and hip girdle. The pain is typically worse in the morning or after periods of inactivity (gelling) and may get better with movement. Because PMR can be associated with giant cell or temporal arteritis, the patient should be queried for temporal headaches, visual changes, and jaw claudication or pain in the muscles of mastication when chewing (17). Examination may reveal tenderness or prominence of the temporal arteries. In patients over 50, one should routinely check laboratory tests, as normal erythrocyte sedimentation rate (ESR) and C-reactive protein (CRP) significantly reduce the likelihood of PMR.

TABLE 1 Differential Diagnosis of Diffuse Arthralgias and Myalgias

Inflammatory
 Polymyalgia rheumatica
 Inflammatory arthritis: rheumatoid arthritis, spondyloarthritidies
 Connective tissues diseases
 Systemic vasculitidies
Infectious
 Hepatitis C
 Human immunodeficiency virus (HIV)
 Lyme disease
 Parvovirus B-19
 Epstein-Barr virus
Noninflammatory
 Degenerative joint/spine disease
 Fibromaylgia
 Myofascial pain syndromes
 Metabolic myopathies
Endocrine
 Hypo- or hyperthyroidism
 Hyperparathyroidism
 Addison's disease
Neurologic diseases
 Multiple sclerosis
 Neuropathic pain
Psychiatric disease
 Major depressive disorder
Drugs
 Statins
 Aromatase inhibitors

Rheumatoid arthritis (RA) should be considered, particularly if the pain complaints are localized to the wrists, metacarpophalangeal joints, proximal interphalangeal joint, or forefoot. The joint-localized pain would typically be accompanied by swelling and warmth, and symptoms should be symmetrical. In RA, joint pain and stiffness would be worse in the morning and last more than 30 minutes, but the patient should be able to describe that joints "loosen up" with activity or after exposure to warm water. If RA is suspected on the basis of this additional history, physical examination should focus on the presence of objective swelling and reduced range of motion, since in patients with FM pain is often difficult to interpret.

More difficult to exclude are seronegative spondyloarthropathies including ankylosing spondylitis, reactive arthritis, psoriatic arthritis, and inflammatory bowel disease–associated arthritis. Symptoms of inflammatory back pain include morning predominance and improvement with exercise. Patients will often complain of buttock pain, which may move from side to side. Of all the inflammatory disorders, spondyloathropathies are the most frequently overlooked in patients with FM-like symptoms (18). If the patient gives a history suggestive of inflammatory back pain, the clinician should evaluate the patient for history of ocular inflammation (e.g., uveiitis), mucosal ulceration, psoriasis, enthesitis (e.g., Achilles tendonitis or plantar fasciitis), dactylitis (e.g., swelling of an entire digit also called "sausage digit"), and symptoms of inflammatory bowel disease. Early sacroiilitis can be difficult to diagnose, and if suspicion for a spondyloarthritis is high and plain films are negative, an MRI may be needed.

The systemic connective tissue diseases (CTDs) in the differential diagnosis of FM are systemic lupus erythematosus (SLE), polymyositis, Sjögren syndrome (SjS), and mixed or undifferentiated CTD. SLE and SjS can be associated with arthalgias, myalgias, and fatigue, which are difficult to distinguish from FM by history alone. Patients should be queried for a history of rash, photosensitivity, mucosal ulcerations, Raynaud's phenomenon, and joint swelling. Patients should be asked about dry mouth and dry eyes, including whether there is crusting in the eyes or a gritty, sandy feeling. It should be clarified as to whether the patient has muscle pain or whether true weakness is present. Any of these findings should trigger the clinician to carefully examine the patient for features of CTD. Furthermore, these findings should prompt antinuclear antibody (ANA) testing. If the patient complains of weakness (e.g., difficulty climbing stairs or styling the hair), measurement of creatine phosphokinase (CPK) and aldolase should be performed. Family history of an autoimmune inflammatory disease can be very helpful in assessing probability for these diseases. If present, a positive family history for any autoimmune disease would strengthen the pretest likelihood for a CTD.

Infectious Etiologies

Infectious etiologies that should most commonly be considered include Lyme disease, parvovirus B-19, HIV, hepatitis B virus (HBV), hepatitis C virus (HCV), and Epstein-Barr virus (19–21). The clinician should take a history to determine if exposure to Lyme disease could have occurred. Clearly, the probability of this disease is increased in certain geographic areas and with outdoor activities. Post-Lyme symptoms include chronic pain and fatigue despite antibiotic treatment in many patients indistinguishable from FM (21,22). Parvovirus B-19 can occur in adults without a rash and should be considered in patients exposed to children. Given the relatively high prevalence of HCV, the clinician should inquire into risk factors for HCV and screen when present. Consideration of HIV and HBV should also occur in at-risk individuals. Epstein-Barr virus infection can also lead to chronic (>3 months) symptoms, though other myotropic viruses are shorter lived. It should be noted that some of these infectious illnesses could also precipitate FM, so consideration may be given to specific treatment for FM if symptoms persist.

Noninflammatory Etiologies

Noninflammatory conditions include FM, myofascial pain syndromes (a more limited musculoskeletal pain syndrome with significant overlap in symptom domains), and generalized osteoarthritis/spondylosis. An occupational history and understanding of any kind of previous trauma or hobbies that entail repetitive motion are particularly important for evaluation of regional musculoskeletal symptoms.

Endocrine disorders, particularly hypo- and hyper-thyroidism but also including parathyroid and adrenal gland dysfunction, can cause widespread myalgias and arthralgias. Vitamin D deficiency is also associated with these symptoms, and questioning the patient about diet and sun exposure followed by screening for at-risk patients is recommended (23,24).

Drug-induced myalgias are seen in patients taking statins and aromatase inhibitors among many others, and a careful history should be able to determine a temporal association between onset of symptoms and the offending drug (25–27).

PHYSICAL EXAMINATION

The physical examination should build from the elements of history and review of systems. Patients presenting with symptoms of widespread pain and fatigue should have a thorough general physical examination. Further physical examination should focus on the musculoskeletal structures; examination of eyes, mucous membranes, skin, and nails should be performed. The clinician should examine the peripheral joints for swelling and range of motion, including joint hypermobility. Particular care should be taken to examine the most painful musculoskeletal sites to determine if common regional disorders such as rotator cuff injuries, bursitis, or osteoarthritis are present. Careful examination of the spine for scoliosis, sacroiliac tenderness, and normal curvature is needed. Neurological examination including muscle strength testing should be performed.

The presence of widespread tenderness is the second critical element of the classification criteria for FM. In practice, this is done by digital palpation of musculotendinous "tender points" (Fig. 2) (1). Palpation is typically performed using the thumb and with a force that causes blanching of the tip of the

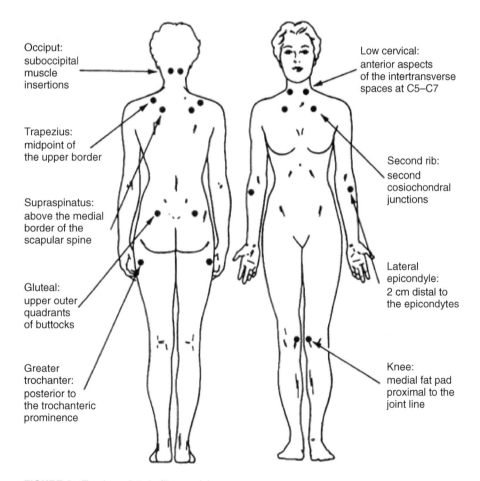

Occiput:
suboccipital
muscle
insertions

Low cervical:
anterior aspects
of the intertransverse
spaces at C5–C7

Trapezius:
midpoint of
the upper border

Second rib:
second
cosiochondral
junctions

Supraspinatus:
above the medial
border of the
scapular spine

Gluteal:
upper outer
quadrants
of buttocks

Lateral
epicondyle:
2 cm distal to
the epicondytes

Greater
trochanter:
posterior to
the trochanteric
prominence

Knee:
medial fat pad
proximal to the
joint line

FIGURE 2   Tender points in fibromyalgia.

examiner's fingernail (approximately 4 kg/cm^2). The research criteria require that 11 of 18 tender points elicit a complaint of pain. Of course, the number of painful tender points is a continuous variable, and the cutoff clearly identifies patients with FM for research purposes. In practice, however, a patient with fewer tender points who also complains of symptoms and syndromes associated with FM is likely to be best conceptualized and treated as having FM.

PERIPHERAL PAIN GENERATORS

The presence of painful musculoskeletal triggers that may contribute to pain and the development of FM should be noted during evaluation (Table 2). It is sometimes useful to initiate treatment of these painful conditions as an initial step to determine if more widespread pain and tenderness persists and will require treatment directed at more central pathways of pain processing. The more clearly the clinician can explain the difference between treatment strategies directed toward pain generators versus central pain processing pathways, the more effectively the patient can contribute to pain management.

LABORATORY AND RADIOGRAPHIC TESTING

Laboratory testing should be guided by history and physical examination. Most patients with a new complaint of chronic widespread pain should be assessed for the most common entities in the differential diagnosis (Table 3). Although

TABLE 2   Peripheral Pain Generators in Fibromyalgia

Osteoarthritis and spondylosis
Other spinal disorders: disk disease, spinal stenosis, scoliosis
Inflammatory arthritis: rheumatoid arthritis, spondyloarthritis (psoriatic arthritis, reactive arthritis, ankylosing spondylitis)
CTDs: systemic lupus erythematosus, Sjogren syndrome, inflammatory myopathies, systemic sclerosis, mixed CTD
Joint hypermobility
Injuries/trauma: whiplash, repetitive strain disorders, bursitis, tendonitis, postsurgical
Myofascial pain disorders: temporomandibular disorders, muscular back pain

Abbreviation: CTD, connective tissue disease.

TABLE 3   Laboratory Testing in Fibromyalgia

Routine
  Erythrocyte sedimentation rate and C-reactive protein
  Complete blood count
  Complete metabolic panel
  Thyroid stimulating hormone
Guided by risk profile
  Hepatitis C
  HIV
  25-OH-vitamin D
Guided by history and physical examination
  Antinuclear antibody
  Anti-SSA and anti-SSB
  Rheumatoid factor and anti-cyclic citrullinated peptide
  Creatine phosphokinase
  Lyme antibody
  Parvovirus B-19 serologies

there is no data to support specific screening laboratories, it is reasonable to screen for inflammatory disorders using ESR and CRP, evaluate for occult inflammatory bowel disease or unexpected hematologic process by complete blood count (CBC), and screen for unexpected endocrine, metabolic, and organ dysfunction with a complete metabolic profile. If there is any concern for SLE, SjS, or polymyositis, one should obtain an ANA. In addition, if dry eyes or dry mouth are present, anti-SSA/Ro and anti-SSB/La may be performed, and if muscle weakness is present, a CPK should be obtained. Laboratory tests for patients with objective joint swelling should include a rheumatoid factor and anti-cyclic citrullinated peptide (anti-CCP). A combination of positive serologies is highly specific for RA (28). Plain radiographs with evidence of erosions can be seen within the first year of symptoms. If RA is suspected and serologies or plain films are negative, other radiographic techniques such as ultrasound or extremity MRI may demonstrate the presence of synovitis. In patients with a strong history suggesting inflammatory back pain, sacroiliac, and lumbosacral spine films should be obtained, and if negative, MRI should be obtained when there is a sufficiently high index of suspicion for a spondyloarthritis. Patients with neck and back pain who have no features suggesting inflammation and no neurologic symptoms should not have imaging procedures.

Because of the high and increasing prevalence of hepatitis C in the population, liver function tests and even specific testing for hepatitis C is increasingly recommended. Screening for other infectious agents is guided by history. Distinguishing hypothyroidism from FM on purely clinical grounds is very difficult, so a thyroid-stimulating hormone (TSH) test should be performed if not done in the past 6 to 12 months. The increasing prevalence of vitamin D deficiency may prompt clinicians to consider screening patients with 25-OH vitamin D levels, particularly if the patient lacks sun exposure and adequate dietary intake.

SUMMARY

Patients presenting with chronic widespread pain, the fellow traveler symptoms of fatigue, sleep disturbance, cognitive dysfunction, anxiety, or depression, and with the presence or history of overlapping conditions should be strongly suspected of having FM. Physical examination could confirm the presence of tenderness. The chief concern is to be certain that the clinician does not miss a triggering or comorbid condition that would require a different treatment approach. A careful history and physical examination along with selected laboratory tests should assure accuracy of the FM diagnosis and should provide confidence that other conditions are identified and addressed.

REFERENCES

1. Wolfe F, Smythe HA, Yunus MB, et al. The American College of Rheumatology 1990 criteria for the classification of fibromyalgia. Arthritis Rheum 1990; 33:160–172.
2. Arnold LM, Crofford LJ, Mease PJ, et al. Patient perspectives on the impact of fibromyalgia. Patient Educ Couns 2008; 73:114–120.
3. Yunus MB, Masi AT, Aldag JC. A controlled study of primary fibromyalgia syndrome: clinical features and association with other functional syndromes. J Rheumatol 1989; 16:62–71.
4. Goldenberg DL, Simms RW, Geiger A, et al. High frequency of fibromyalgia in patients with chronic fatigue seen in a primary care practice. Arthritis Rheum 1990; 33:381–387.

5. Glass JM. Cognitive dysfunction in fibromyalgia and chronic fatigue syndrome: new trends and future directions. Curr Rheumatol Rep 2006; 8:425–429.
6. Glass JM, Park DC, Minear M, et al. Memory beliefs and function in fibromyalgia patients. J Psychosom Res 2005; 58:263–269.
7. Arnold LM, Crofford LJ, Martin SA, et al. The effect of anxiety and depression on improvements in pain in a randomized, controlled trial of pregabalin for treatment of fibromyalgia. Pain Med 2007; 8:633–638.
8. Aaron LA, Buchwald D. A review of the evidence for overlap among unexplained clinical conditions. Ann Intern Med 2001; 134:868–881.
9. Marcus DA, Bernstein C, Rudy TE. Fibromyalgia and headache: an epidemiologic study supporting migraine as part of the fibromyalgia syndrome. Clin Rheumatol 2005; 24:595–601.
10. Korszun A, Papadopoulos E, Demitrack M, et al. The relationship between temporomandibular disorders and stress-associated syndromes. Oral surg Oral Med Oral Pathol Oral Radiol Endod 1998; 86:416–420.
11. Drossman DA, Corazziari E, Talley NJ, et al. The functional gastrointestinal disorders. Diagnosis, pathophysiology and treatment: a multinational consensus. 2nd ed. McLean, VA: Degnon Associates, 2000.
12. Hanno PM, Landis JR, Matthews-Cook Y, et al. The diagnosis of interstitial cystitis revisited: lessons learned from the National Institutes of Health Interstitial Cystitis Database Study. J Urol 1999; 161:553–557.
13. Twiss C, Kilpatrick L, Craske M, et al. Increased startle responses in interstitial cystitis: evidence for central hyperresponsiveness to visceral related threat. J Urol 2009; 181:2127–2133.
14. Naliboff BD, Waters AM, Labus JS, et al. Increased acoustic startle responses in IBS patients during abdominal and nonabdominal threat. Psychosom Med 2008; 70: 920–927.
15. Crofford LJ, Demitrack MA. Evidence that abnormalities of central neurohormonal systems are key to understanding fibromylagia and chronic fatigue syndrome. Rheum Dis Clin North Am 1996; 22:267–284.
16. Roy-Burne P, Smith WR, Goldberg J, et al. Post-traumatic stress disorder among patients with chronic pain and chronic fatigue. Psychol Med 2004; 34:363–368.
17. Seo P, Stone JH. Large-vessel vasculitis. Arthritis Rheum 2004; 15:128–139.
18. Fitzcharles MA, Esdaile JM. The overdiagnosis of fibromyalgia syndrome. Am J Med 1997; 103:44–50.
19. Buskila D, Atzeni F, Sarzi-Puttini P. Etiology of fibromyalgia: the possible role of infection and vaccination. Autoimmun Rev 2008; 8:41–43.
20. Vassilopoulos D, Calabrese LH. Virally associated arthritis 2008: clinical, epidemiologic, and pathophysiologic considerations. Arthritis Res Ther 2008; 10:215.
21. Cairns V, Godwin J. Post-Lyme borreliosis syndrome: a meta-analysis of reported symptoms. Int J Epidemiol 2005; 34:1340–1345.
22. Dinerman H, Steere AC. Lyme disease associated with fibromyalgia. Ann Intern Med 1992; 117:281–285.
23. Atherton K, Berry DJ, Parsons T, et al. Vitamin D and chronic widespread pain in a white middle-aged British population: evidence from a cross-sectional population survey. Ann Rheum Dis 2008 [Epub ahead of print].
24. Turner MK, Hooten WM, Schmidt JE, et al. Prevalence and clinical correlates of vitamin D inadequacy among patients with chronic pain. Pain Med 2008; 9:979–984
25. Felson DT, Cummings SR. Aromatase inhibitors and the syndrome of arthralgias with estrogen deprivation. Arthritis Rheum 2005; 52:2594–2598.
26. Presant CA, Bosserman L, Young T, et al. Aromatase inhibitor-associated arthralgia and/or bone pain: frequency and characterization in non-clinical trial patients. Clin Breast Cancer 2007; 7:775–778.
27. Jacobson TA. Toward "pain-free" statin prescribing: clinical algorithm for diagnosis and management of myalgia. Mayo Clin Proc 2008; 83:687–700.
28. Ateş A, Karaaslan Y, Aksaray S. Predictive value of antibodies to cyclic citrullinated peptide in patients with early arthritis. Clin Rheumatol 2007; 26:499–504.

3

Nonpharmacological, Complementary and Alternative Treatments for Fibromyalgia

Robert Alan Bonakdar
Scripps Center for Integrative Medicine, Scripps Clinic, La Jolla, California, U.S.A.

INTRODUCTION AND OVERVIEW

Fibromyalgia (FM) has been recently described as "a common, poorly understood condition with limited treatment options" (1). Thus, it is no surprise that nonpharmacological treatments, including complementary and alternative medicine (CAM), are common choices for FM patients looking at ways to manage their condition. The following (chapter 4) will provide an overview of these treatment options, including prevalence, patient rationale for utilization and clinical efficacy. Most importantly, as many of these choices are accessed without the input of a clinician, the chapter hopes to provide guidance regarding the discussion and coordination of care for these treatments. This chapter will not focus on the use of traditional exercise or psychological interventions that are covered elsewhere in the book.

Overview and Prevalence

Nonpharmacological and CAM treatments include a vast array of choices for the FM patient. The definitions for these treatments vary and are constantly being updated. Nonpharmacological treatments are typically defined as options that are not prescription medications. However, several options that have been nonprescription options in the past, such as omega-3 oils or B-vitamins, are now available in formulations requiring a prescription. In addition, several options, such as S-adenosyl methionine (SAMe), which are nonprescription in the United States, may require prescriptions outside the United States. Similarly, CAM was previously defined as treatments not included in medical school training. Currently, more than 60% of the nation's allopathic medical schools are providing some level of instruction on CAM (2). More recently, CAM has been defined by the National Institutes of Health Center for Complementary and Alternative Medicine (NCCAM) as treatments or medical systems that are not typically incorporated in conventional treatment recommendations. This definition has evolved to include integrative medicine, which is the practice of incorporating selected evidence-based CAM options into mainstream practice (3). The NCCAM system classifies CAM into categories, which are helpful for discussion. Currently, there is no consensus and large overlap over these terms. For this chapter the nonpharmacological and CAM treatments reviewed will be referred to collectively as NP/CAM. An overview of NP/CAM categorized under NCCAM headings is noted in Table 1.

Prevalence of NP/CAM Use

NP/CAM use is quite common, especially in those suffering from pain. CAM usage was reported in approximately a third of the U.S. population in 1990 and increased to 42% by 1997. At that point this represented 628 million office visits

TABLE 1 Overview of Nonpharmacological and Complementary and Alternative Medicine Treatments

Category overview	Examples	
1. Alternative medical systems Systems of care based on unifying health paradigms that may incorporate individual treatments including those noted in the categories below.	Traditional Chinese Medicine Ayurveda Naturopathy Homeopathy	
2. Mind-body interventions Diverse techniques that utilized cognitive, behavioral, and movement therapies to modify and increase awareness between mental and physiological functioning.	Biofeedback Meditation Yoga Exercise, various tai chi/Qigong Creative therapies (art, music, or dance) Relaxation	Hypnosis Visualization Guided imagery Cognitive-behavioral therapies Group support Autogenic training Spirituality
3. Biologically Based Therapies Therapies that modify nutrient intake either through dietary intervention or supplementation	Dietary modification (dietary elimination, fasting, or specific dietary regimen) Dietary supplements: Herbal supplements (white willow bark) Nonherbal supplements (glucosamine), vitamins (vitamin D), minerals (selenium)	
4. Manipulative and body-based methods Techniques that utilize manipulation, movement and/or stretching of one or more parts of the body.	Chiropractic manipulation Osteopathic manipulation Manual and massage therapy	
5. Energy therapies (biofield therapies) Techniques that involve the application of human or nonhuman energy fields.	Acupuncture Qigong Healing touch Therapeutic touch	

Source: Adapted from Ref. 3.

and $27 million spent on CAM services, which far exceeded total out-of-pocket expenditure and office visits (328 million) for conventional primary care providers in the same year. A follow-up analysis demonstrated that approximately one-third of the visits to CAM providers were for the treatment of musculoskeletal pain (4). A more recent analysis of CAM use by the National Institutes of Health (NIH) found that most of the top 10 reasons for CAM use were related to musculoskeletal complaints (5).

When focused on rheumatologic diagnoses, including FM, the utilization of NP/CAM appears to be even more prevalent. In one survey, CAM use by patients with FM was significantly higher than in the comparison group without FM (56% versus 21%) (6). Compared with other rheumatologic diagnoses, FM patients tend to be the most regular users of CAM. In comparing FM patients with non-FM rheumatology patients, one survey found FM patients with a higher level of CAM use including overall use (91% vs. 63%), over-the-counter products (70% vs. 54%), spiritual practices (48% vs. 37%), and visits to alternative practitioners (26% vs. 12%). Of note, two-thirds of FM patients had utilized multiple CAM modalities concomitantly. This makes the coordination of care quite challenging as discussed below (7).

Predictors and Patterns of Use
Those with FM who utilize CAM have similarities to the general CAM utilizer. Namely, those with FM who use CAM are more likely to be women with higher levels of education and income. Their clinical status appears to be poorer as indicated by greater duration and severity of pain and comorbidities with overall higher levels of disability (8). Those using CAM have health values, beliefs, and coping systems that are also quite important to keep in mind. Those who are involved in "active coping behaviors," which include physical activity and particular diets, tend to view CAM use in a similar manner (9). Also those with a more "holistic outlook" wish to utilize complementary methods that take their viewpoint into consideration (10).

There has been speculation that CAM use signals dissatisfaction with conventional care. One survey found that rheumatology patients with more medical skepticism had a higher likelihood of utilizing a CAM provider. This finding was especially true for FM patients (11). However, the more likely scenario is that of CAM as an adjunct to conventional care. In fact, dissatisfaction with conventional care did not predict use of CAM in a previous survey and less than 5% of CAM users did so in isolation from conventional care. Most CAM users state that their motivations for CAM use provide more control over their healthcare, and up to 80% reported benefit from its use in a previous survey (9). In addition, CAM users have been noted to have more frequent relationships with a primary care physician, have regular physician follow-up and good compliance with recommended preventative health behaviors such as regular mammography (12). Thus what may be termed medical skepticism may in fact be an active coping behavior attempting to identify and incorporate potentially helpful treatments. As discussed below, the coordination of these efforts by a medical provider is quite important to help maximize treatment utility.

Types of Treatments Utilized
Because of the prevalence of CAM use, clinicians seeing FM patients are likely to encounter a majority of the treatments outlined in Table 1 when reviewing patient histories. In a previous survey of NP/CAM use, there was a 98% prevalence of these strategies and the most common used on a daily basis included exercise, bed rest, dietary supplements, heat treatment, and spirituality/praying (8). Another Internet survey of over 2500 FM patients found that the most commonly utilized and beneficial treatments were rest, heat modalities, prayer, massage, and pool therapy. Other NP/CAM treatments utilized but with less perceived efficacy included dietary supplements, relaxation/meditation, massage/reflexology, manipulation, counseling and cognitive-behavioral therapy (CBT), physical therapy, transcutaneous electrical nerve stimulation (TENS), acupuncture, support groups, pilates, energy healing (reiki and healing touch), biofeedback, and hypnosis (13).

Expenditure
The cost burden of FM care has been discussed because of the large number of treatments utilized by patients. In a survey of insured FM patients, those who used CAM had more provider visits than FM patients not using CAM. However, as expenditure per visit for CAM visits was lower than for non-CAM visits, FM

patient who were using CAM had similar expenditures as CAM nonusers (6). These authors postulate "... CAM providers may offer an economic alternative for patients with FM syndrome (FMS) seeking symptomatic relief." Overall, the cost of FM care appears to be less as predicted by CAM use than by level of disability, with one survey noting a 20% cost increase with each additional comorbid condition (14).

APPROACH TO THE PATIENT

Regardless of their experience or particular beliefs about CAM, clinicians have an ethical obligation to discuss treatment alternatives with their FM patients. This is quite pertinent in the FM population that has an especially high use of NP/CAM. In this setting, it is especially important to have an open, nonjudgmental discussion about all treatments being considered or utilized to provide full and optimal coordination of care. Unfortunately, the interaction between patients and clinicians regarding CAM use is often suboptimal. This situation is linked to several factors noted below including patient and clinician CAM knowledge base, level of discussion, and management strategies that include charting and follow-up. Several strategies and pertinent resources are reviewed to help optimize the approach to the FM patient.

Knowledge Base

The knowledge base of the average clinician and consumer regarding NP/CAM is suboptimal including popular areas such as dietary supplements. Physician surveys have found that physicians may have an insufficient general understanding of commonly utilized supplements as well as their safety, regulation, and interaction profiles (15,16). Similarly, consumers and patients tend to have misconceptions regarding product claims and efficacy. As pointed out by a previous Harris Poll, majority of consumers believe that the government ensures a higher level of safety and regulation than actually exists (17). These misconceptions as well as biased or anecdotal information found on some health websites and advertising may create a scenario of decreased perceived need for clinician guidance regarding CAM (18).

Discussion

The level of discussion regarding NP-CAM that occurs in the average pain consultation can be quite minimal. This is exemplified by the example of an editorial from the journal *Pain*, titled "Food and pain: Should we be more interested in what our patients eat?" The average pain clinician does not spend significant time discussing diet in general or as an intervention. The reasons for this may include lack of training and resources and more comfort prescribing other interventions including medication (19,20). The level of discussion regarding CAM specifically may be even more deficient. Surveys have found that in approximately 70% of encounters there was no discussion of CAM use in which neither the patient nor the clinician introduced the topic (21). More concerning is the fact that if a patient is hospitalized by a specialist, CAM use is not identified up to 88% of the time (22).

It is important to understand why patients may not discuss CAM use. Surveys indicate that factors including anticipation of a negative clinician response as well as belief that the clinician will not provide useful information motivated nondiscussion (23). However, most important may be clinician inquiry, because patients demonstrate a willingness to disclose supplements use, but only if asked by a clinician (24). Unfortunately, a recent survey of physicians found that few felt comfortable discussing CAM with their patients. One of the major reasons for this lack of comfort was related to a need for improved knowledge base regarding CAM (84% of responders). It is theorized that with improved education and knowledge base about CAM, physicians may be more willing to discuss and counsel patients (25).

Patient and Clinician Education

A number of resources are available to clinicians interested in better understanding of NP/CAM as a means of improving patient communication and treatment options. These resources are listed in Table 2 and include print and online information on evidence-based use of NP/CAM as well as continuing

TABLE 2   Selected NP/CAM Resources for the Clinician

Internet

- The Arthritis Foundation (http://www.arthritis.org). Finding education, exercise, and support services for FM patients.
- The National Center for Complementary and Alternative Medicine (NCCAM) (http://nccam.nih.gov). Overview of CAM fields as well as information on clinical trials and patient education materials.
- CAM on PubMed (www.nlm.nih.gov/medlineplus/alternativemedicine.html). Focused search on PubMed for articles with a focus on alternative and complementary medicine.
- Cochrane Library (www.cochrane.org). Collection of systematic reviews with a complementary medicine field.
- NIH Office of Dietary Supplements and International Bibliographic Information on Dietary Supplements (IBIDS) (http://ods.od.nih.gov). Collaborative database of available abstract on dietary supplements.
- FDA Division of Dietary Supplement (http://vm:cfsan.fda.gov/~dms/supplmnt/html). Discussion of dietary supplement regulation including list of recalls and warnings.
- Natural Medicines Comprehensive Database (www.naturaldatabase.com). An extensive collection of supplement information including uses, indication, efficacy, and adverse effects with a drug interactions checker.
- National FM Association (http://www.fmaware.org).
- Longwood Herbal Taskforce (www.mcp.edu/herbal). Collection of clinically oriented monographs and reviewed Internet link.

Peer-reviewed resources for patients

- MedlinePlus (www.nlm.nih.gov/medlineplus/alternativemedicine.html). Patient-oriented summary of Medline published research and international health news.
- The National Center for Complementary and Alternative Medicine (NCCAM) (www.nccam.nih.gov). NIH clearinghouse of government funded initiatives in CAM including research, fellowships, grants, and patient education materials.
- Natural Medicine Comprehensive Database patient handouts (www.naturaldatabase.com).
- The Arthritis Foundation (http://www.arthritis.org) that offers a number of resource in the nonpharmacological/CAM area, including section on
  - Working with your doctor and complementary medicine
  - What complementary medicine might do for you
  - Supplement guide
- Dietary Guidelines (www.MyPyramid.gov)
  - http://www.mypyramid.gov offers personalized eating plans, interactive tools to help you plan and assess your food choices, and advice to help you.
- Exercise guidelines: FM Information Foundation (FIF)
  - http://www.myalgia.com

TABLE 3   The H.E.R.B.A.L. Mnemonic © Robert Bonakdar

Hear the patient out with respect
Educate the patient
Record
Be aware of potential interaction and side effects
Agree to discuss and follow-up
Learn

Source: From Ref. 26.

medical education courses available to clinicians. The H.E.R.B.A.L. Mnemonic is offered in Table 3 as a clinical tool for aiding clinicians when discussing and managing CAM use, especially dietary supplements.

REGULATION

The regulation of NP/CAM varies widely based on the therapy described, the training of practitioners, and the state laws. For example, acupuncture provided by a licensed acupuncturist (LAc) or physician acupuncturist may have vastly differing regulation as set forth by the state board of Traditional Chinese Medicine, medical board, or department of consumer affairs. In addition, the level of training, oversight, and continuing education for acupuncture vary widely by state, and the referring clinician should help guide patients in finding qualified and experienced CAM practitioners whenever possible. Verification of licensure can be obtained by contacting the state's medical board, department of consumer affairs, or therapy-specific national certification organizations as listed in Table 4.

Dietary supplements are regulated according to the Dietary Supplement Health and Education Act (DSHEA) of 1994. Regulation differs from prescription medication, which must proceed through multiphase trials to gain approval from the Food and Drug Administration (FDA). Supplements (with established ingredients) are not strictly required to have safety, efficacy, or bioavailability data prior to marketing. The FDA must utilize adverse drug reports and product analysis to monitor products in the marketplace (27,28). Two more recent regulatory measures—The Dietary Supplement and Nonprescription Drug Consumer Protection Act (S. 3546), which mandates the reporting of serious adverse events to the FDA, and Good Manufacturing Practices (GMPs) for dietary supplements, which began incorporation in August of 2007—should be helpful in ensuring better regulated supplements (29).

In addition to the above governmental measures, several agencies offer testing and monitoring services that allow manufacturers to demonstrate their adherence to regulatory standards. Those that pass inspection may carry an independent "Seal of

TABLE 4   Regulation Resources for Complementary and Alternative Medicine

Organization/agency	Website
Federation of State Medical Boards	http://www.fsmb.org/m_pub.html
American Academy of Medical Acupuncture	http://www.medicalacupuncture.org
The National Certification Commission for Acupuncture and Oriental Medicine	http://www.nccaom.org/
American Chiropractic Association's	http://www.acatoday.org
The National Certification Board for Therapeutic Massage and Bodywork	http://www.ncbtmb.com
Association of Accredited Naturopathic Colleges	www.aanmc.org

TABLE 5 Government and Independent Regulatory Agencies

Agency	Website/contact information
Government	
Food and Drug Administration (FDA) Medwatch Program for collecting adverse reactions to prescription and OTC medications as well as dietary supplements	www.fda.gov/medwatch
Federal Trade Commission (FTC) site for submitting complaints on false or misleading advertising	www.ftc.gov/ftc/complaint.htm
American Association of Poison Control Centers for reporting and management of adverse effects	www.poison.org or (800)222-1222
Independent labs providing supplement testing	
The Consumerlab Product Review	www.Consumerlab.com
Dietary Supplement Verification Program (DSVP) through the United States Pharmacopeia (USP)	www.uspverified.org
National Sanitation Foundation (NSF)	www.NSF.ORG/consumer/ dietary_supplements

Approval" on their label and advertising. Several of the government and independent agencies currently involved in oversight are listed in Table 5. Clinicians should become familiar with well-regulated and well-researched brands for the supplements that are most likely to be discussed with patients.

INTERVENTIONS: EVIDENCE-GUIDED CARE

FM patients encounter, consider, and incorporate a large number of interventions for their condition and comorbidities. Understanding the motivation for, benefit from, and integrative potential for these treatments on an individual basis is key in helping to frame an effective multidisciplinary treatment plan. Unfortunately, the research basis in this area is quite heterogeneous and at time difficult to interpret. As an example, a previous systematic review of non-pharmacological interventions for FM examined 25 randomized trials in the areas of education, exercise, physical and hydrotherapy, relaxation therapy, CBT, and acupuncture. Overall, the methodological quality of studies appeared fairly low with typically small subject sizes. Because of the wide range of methodology, intervention, and outcome measures, the reviewers had difficulty in drawing any conclusions and did not find strong evidence for any single intervention. Although moderate evidence of aerobic exercise was noted, the researchers noted a need for larger and more rigorous trials (30).

While awaiting more definitive evidence-based guidelines in this area, the clinician needs to provide evidence-guided care. In the setting of FM, because of the varied number of intervention and methodologies, the provider must many times strive for evidence-guided care to find a successful compromise between available clinical evidence, patient preference, and clinical experience. In this paradigm, the clinician must review the available evidence to determine the safety and efficacy of various interventions. This is especially true of interventions that may be provided and initiated with varied methodologies, dosages, and directives. A prime example of this is acupuncture for FM, which is covered in more detail below.

If a clinician were to follow the conclusion of a recent meta-analysis in this area when encountering a refractory FM patient interested in trying this

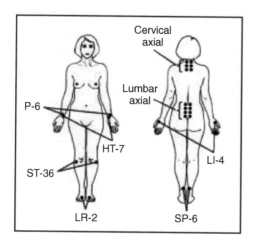

FIGURE 1 Acupuncture protocol from randomized trial in FM. *Source*: From Ref. 40.

intervention, his or her response may be to avoid this intervention. However, when more closely examined, not all interventions were similar, and all of the positive trials utilized electroacupuncture. Further evaluation would identify a clear, standardized protocol utilized in a positive trial from the Mayo Clinic that may be appropriate to recommend (Fig. 1).

In the setting of acupuncture or any NP/CAM if there are no positive trials and/or the treatment demonstrates significant potential for harm then the directive should be one of avoidance. However, if the treatment is of minimal harm and has the potential of benefit (such as guided imagery) or has positive evidence that demands a more focused detail of the intervention (see acupuncture below), it may be recommended. This recommendation requires attention to specific protocols for modalities and specific dosage and brand for supplements along with appropriate monitoring and follow-up reassessment after a trial period. Figure 2 provides a potential framework for stepwise, evidence-guided incorporation of NP/CAM options in FM.

As several recent reviews of FM treatment point out, it is important to keep in mind both pharmacological and nonpharmacological treatment options that approach the pain of FM as well as the complex web of comorbidities (31,32). As the EULAR (European League Against Rheumatism) recommendations for FM management, which examined 39 pharmacological and 59 nonpharmacological interventions, noted:

> Optimal treatment requires a multidisciplinary approach with a combination of non-pharmacological and pharmacological treatment modalities tailored according to pain intensity, function, associated features, such as depression, fatigue and sleep disturbance, in discussion with the patient. (33)

Treatment Overview

Acupuncture

Acupuncture typically involves the therapeutic insertion of fine needles at selected body points based on a traditional or neuroanatomical basis. It is often utilized in the setting of FM because it is believed to be helpful for pain management based on specific and nonspecific local, neurochemical, and cortical

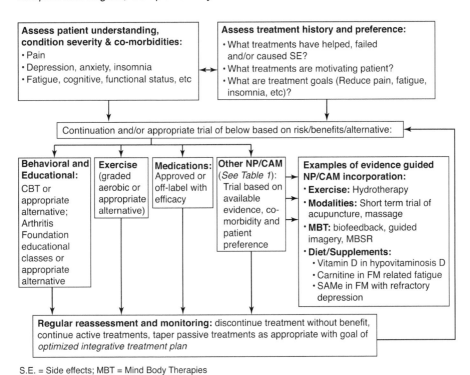

FIGURE 2 Fibromyalgia: An integrative evidence-guided approach.

S.E. = Side effects; MBT = Mind Body Therapies

modulation (34,35). The potential for benefit in the setting of FM is difficult to answer largely based on the poor methodology and varied application of acupuncture in trials (36). As an example, a previous review of these trials found that only one was graded as high quality. In this randomized trial of 70 FM patients, electroacupuncture outperformed sham electroacupuncture in the majority of outcome measure (37). The reviewers noted that the "limited amount of high-quality evidence suggests that real acupuncture is more effective than sham acupuncture for improving symptoms of patients with FMS." More recently, an analysis of five trials in which three were positive (all electroacupuncture) and two negative concluded that heterogeneity and varied methodological strength of current evidence did not support the use of acupuncture (38). These conclusions have been questioned due to the partial treatment effect of control interventions (off-sight or superficial needling), which in the FM population may not be completely inert (39).

In reviewing the evidence, one of the better-controlled trials of acupuncture demonstrating benefit in FM came from the Mayo Clinic. In this trial, patients were randomized and in blinded fashion provided with six standardized acupuncture treatments over three weeks (protocol utilized is noted in Fig. 1) (40). The trial demonstrated improvement in FIQ as well as fatigue and anxiety scores with real versus sham acupuncture. Thus from evidence-guided standpoint as discussed earlier, acupuncture appears safe and efficacious in selected protocols such as that described in the Mayo Clinic trial. In patients interested in this intervention, care should be taken to recommend a trusted provider who will be able to follow available recommendation and protocols to optimize the potential benefit of this intervention. Recommendation for all NP/ CAM should also include regular follow-up for reevaluation, which includes continuing or tapering treatment as appropriate as well as coordinating with other care options.

Physical Therapies
Modalities and physical therapies include a wide range of therapies that are practitioner based and/or patient guided. Exercise overview is provided elsewhere in the book and is only covered in this chapter when provided in conjunction with other therapies or related to CAM (tai chi, yoga). The most common of these therapies utilized in FM are reviewed below. These therapies are based on several potential areas of benefit, which may correct areas of abnormality seen in FM including decreased microcirculation (41), peripheral blood flow (42), physical conditioning, and endurance.

Hydrotherapy and Balneotherapy
Heated pool therapy (i.e., balneotherapy) is recognized as a helpful traditional treatment of FM. In many trials, land-based exercise of some type is included with the balneotherapy making differentiation difficult. However, the majority of balneotherapy-only trials continue to demonstrate benefit in functional status and pain (43,44). In addition, a more recent comparison found both aquatic therapy and home-based exercise programs to be beneficial in typical FM end points including pain and functional ability, but found that aquatic therapy was best able to maintain improvement, including pain reduction, at week 24 (45). A recent systematic review of 10 trials found strong evidence that hydrotherapy was effective in improving health status, tender point count, and pain level in patients with FM (46). Because of the consistent research benefit of hydrotherapy for FM symptoms, its low cost, and minimal likelihood for dropout, it should be recommended freely by clinicians. Clinicians can use resources, such as the Arthritis Foundation as noted in the Table 2, to help identify locations for heated pool therapy for their patients.

Low-Level Laser Therapy
Low-level laser therapy (LLLT) refers to the application of low-intensity monochromatic, typically nonthermal, wavelengths of light for therapeutic benefit. Although LLLT has been used for several decades in Europe, the mechanism for LLLT has not been fully elucidated but appears to be a photochemical cellular reaction that may improve tissue parameters such as local microcirculation. In the setting of FM, LLLT appears quite attractive in that it may provide a noninvasive modality to approach the potential microcirculation and peripheral blood flow dysfunction. Several small studies have been done specifically in an FM population. In a study of 75 FM subjects, a galliumarsenide (Ga-As) laser treatment [3 minutes or $2\,J/cm^2$ at each tender point daily $\times$ 10 days] was compared to placebo laser or 10 mg amitriptyline at bedtime. Both active groups improved significantly with the laser group noting better pain and fatigue scores and the medication group noting more improvement in morning stiffness and depression scores after therapy (47).

A second randomized study ($N = 40$) by the same authors evaluated LLLT in female subjects with FM (48). Subjects received LLLT similar to the protocol above or placebo laser daily for two weeks. The laser group demonstrated significant improvement observed in pain, muscle spasm, morning stiffness, and tender point numbers versus sham laser ($p < 0.05$). No side effects were reported. In a third pilot study ($N = 20$), adding LLLT to a stretching program did not provide any additional benefit beyond stretching alone (49). Although initial research favors the use of LLLT in FM, additional larger trials with longer follow-up using varying laser parameters are encouraged. At this point, for patients enquiring about the use of LLLT, they should be told that only preliminary evidence from short-term trials using a laser at the specification above is available.

Magnetic Stimulation: Static, Pulsed, and Transcranial

Several studies have attempted to evaluate the use of static magnets in the setting of FM. Although some studies have shown short-term benefits, especially with the use of an electromagnetic shielding fabric, most have not demonstrated benefit beyond sham magnets or usual care group (50,51). Pulsed electromagnetic fields (PEMFs) generate deeper penetration and possibly a central effect as noted in animal studies. Two small ($N < 20$) randomized studies have demonstrated pain reduction versus placebo in patients exposed to varying duration of PEMF (400 μT) (52,53). The most promising area of magnetic research has focused on repetitive transcranial magnetic stimulation (rTMS). Several small trials have noted significant central effects, including modulation of the motor cortex (M1), which has provided short to moderate length benefit in pain and functional status, especially sleep dysfunction (54,55). Initial data are quite promising and additional trials are pending to elucidate safety and length of benefit from treatment.

Electrical Stimulation

Various types of TENS devices have been utilized in the setting of FM. Unfortunately there have been few randomized controlled trial (RCT) in this area, making it hard to draw any conclusions (56). Because of cutaneous hypersensitivity, most physical therapy modalities for FM focus on less invasive (LLLT) and more palatable (hydrotherapy, magnetic stimulation) interventions. One exception in this area may be microcurrent electrical stimulation that utilizes subthreshold stimulation at local or reflex sites (such as biauricular stimulation). There have been several small trials that demonstrate tolerability and short-term benefit in the setting of pain and sleep status in FM patients (57,58).

Massage Therapy

Massage therapy is a common treatment choice for FM patients with several trials attempting to examine its efficacy in the setting of FM pain and symptoms. Two small trials found massage beneficial in FM-related pain, anxiety, and insomnia as compared to TENS or relaxation therapy (59,60). Other trials have found either no benefit or benefit that reduced over time (70% residual benefit at 3 months and 10% residual benefit at 6 months) as may be expected from a passive therapy (61,62). Overall, the research on massage is heterogeneous but appears to point to short-term benefit in selected patients. Massage may be considered by a qualified practitioner familiar with FM if other physical therapies have failed. Patients should be made aware of its passive nature and they should utilize short-term gains to transition to more active management approaches.

Mind-Body Therapies

Mind-body therapies (MBTs) are diverse techniques that utilize cognitive, behavioral, and movement therapies to modify and increase awareness between mental and physiological functioning. Traditional psychological interventions are discussed elsewhere in the book. The following section focuses primarily on less traditional MBTs often considered by patients. Hadhazy et al. reviewed 13 trials, including 7 trials receiving a high methodological score, involving 802 subjects (63). They found that compared to waiting list/treatment as usual, MBTs show strong evidence of being more effective for self-efficacy and limited evidence for improving quality of life. Compared to placebo, MBTs were more effective for pain and global improvement. There was no conclusive evidence that MBT was more effective than other therapies utilized, such as physiotherapy, psychotherapy, or education/attention control for all outcomes. Interestingly, moderate-/high-intensity exercise had strong evidence that it was more effective for pain and physical function than MBT. However, MBT plus exercise has moderate evidence that it is more effective than usual care or wait list for self-efficacy and quality of life.

Education/Self-Guided Treatments

Because the etiology, diagnosis, and treatment of FM are often misunderstood, proper education and self-management approaches are essential. Several trials have incorporated education or Internet-based self-management programs and found that they may provide an important component of overall treatment. As an example, in a large trial of arthritis subjects, including FM patients, an Internet-based course demonstrated significant improvement in four of six health status measures as well as self-efficacy as compared to controls after one year (64). In a large, well-designed trial by Rooks et al., participants were randomized to possible exercise as well as 7 two-hour education sessions, which were at two-week intervals. The educational component utilized the FM Self-Help Course (FSHC) that explains the condition as well as self-management skills for dealing with symptoms and increasing functional status. Although education component did not provide significant benefit alone, the combination of education with exercise made significant gains (beyond exercise alone) that were sustained for six months (1).

Cognitive-Behavioral Therapies

CBTs enable patients to better understand how various beliefs, thoughts, and perceptions can affect their condition. Techniques such as restructuring, prioritization, and goal setting are utilized to repattern behavior. In the setting of FM, a number of preliminary or noncontrolled trials have found benefit with the use of CBT (64–67). Although better trials are needed to more fully endorse CBT in FM, the available evidence provides reason to believe that this therapy can be helpful in FM and has strong evidence in several areas of typical FM comorbidity such as depression. This intervention should be recommended, especially in patients who exhibit psychological sequelae as a means of better approaching their condition or other therapies. (For further details regarding psychological interventions, including CBT please see chapters 5 and 8.)

Biofeedback

Biofeedback utilized various techniques or sensors to increase mind-body awareness and identify areas of potential modification such as muscle tension (sEMG) or autonomic tone [peripheral temperature, heart rate variability (HRV), galvanic skin response]. Because of the autonomic dysfunction described in FM, biofeedback training affords a potential treatment for active nervous system retraining (68). Most trials in this area have been small but demonstrate benefit with various approaches including a pilot study demonstrating decreased depression and pain and improvement in functional status from initiation to three-month follow-up in FM subjects utilizing HRV biofeedback (69). Several studies have demonstrated synergistic benefit from the use of biofeedback with other approaches, possibly by increasing awareness and decreasing autonomic overarousal. As an example, 119 FM subjects were randomly assigned to biofeedback/relaxation training, exercise training, a combination treatment, or an attention control program. All three active groups improved in functional self-efficacy with the combination group most able to maintain gains made at two years (70).

Mindfulness-Based Stress Reduction and Meditation

Meditation and more comprehensive approaches, such as the mindfulness-based stress reduction (MBSR) programs, which provide multidimensional mind-body approaches focusing on awareness to manage chronic conditions, have been investigated in the setting of FM. Initial studies found that group mindfulness meditation training programs were effective in reducing symptoms and maintaining benefit, including anxiety and panic in the majority of participants as well as maintaining these reductions at three-month follow-up (71,72). More recently a controlled trial utilizing an eight-week MBSR intervention for depression in 91 FM subjects demonstrated significant improvement in symptoms versus control, which was maintained at two-month follow-up (73). The strongest evidence comes from a recent trial that examined an eight-week MBSR intervention versus active social support with a three-year follow-up. MBSR intervention provided significantly greater benefits than the control intervention in pain, QoL subscales, coping with pain, anxiety, depression, and somatic complaints that were maintained at three-year follow-up (74).

Guided Imagery

Guided imagery appears to be a simple, active treatment, especially in potentially improving self-efficacy and functional status in FM. A six-week guided imagery intervention demonstrated significant improvement in FIQ scores and ratings of self-efficacy for managing pain while not changing pain as measured by the SF-MPQ (Short-form McGill Pain Questionnaire) (75). A small trial comparing "pleasant imagery" versus amitriptyline in a one-month trial found significant pain reduction with the imagery and no significant change with medication versus usual care at one month (76). Of note, there is additional support for the use of guided imagery in the setting of comorbidities often seen with FM such as interstitial cystitis (77). Thus the clinician should readily recommend guided imagery especially in the setting of FM patients with high comorbidities and high likelihood for compliance with a daily guided imagery session.

Movement-Based MBTs: tai chi, Qigong, and Yoga

The benefits of exercise cannot be underestimated in the setting of FM. These may include reducing obesity (which has been linked to poorer quality of life and pain status), as well as improving fatigue, mood, and physical/cardiovascular endurance (78). For a complete discussion of exercise please refer to chapter 7. "Mindful exercise" is a term often referring to gentle movement-based therapies that have an appreciable level of mind-body awareness. These therapies include, but are not limited to, tai chi, Qigong, and yoga. The awareness component of these therapies may have additional benefits in improving autonomic dysfunction and may be especially attractive for patients who are particularly interested in incorporating these therapies or who may not be able to incorporate traditional exercise therapies.

A pilot study of 39 FM subjects who performed a one-hour tai chi routine twice weekly for six weeks noted improvement in the FIQ and the Short Form-36 (SF-36) (79). A more recent randomized trial of a seven-week Qigong intervention in 57 subjects with FMS noted improvement in pain and psychological well-being. These benefits were maintained at four-month follow-up (80). Yoga has also been utilized in preliminary trials including a trial of 40 women with FM randomized to yoga (emphasizing stretching, breathing, and relaxing) or yoga plus Tui Na massage for eight weeks. Both groups demonstrated significant improvement in the fibromyalgia impact questionnaire (FIQ) and visual analogue scale (VAS) scores after the intervention. Interestingly the Tui Na massage group demonstrated lower pain scores during treatment but the yoga-only group maintained greater improvement at follow-up, possibly showing longer-term benefit for more active treatment versus passive techniques (81).

Several other trials in this area have noted equivocal results versus controls or standard therapy (82,83). Because of methodological weakness including small size and high dropout rates, definitive conclusions regarding these therapies are difficult. However, mindful exercise appears to offer a safe alternative for patients who have either failed other activity approaches or who are especially motivated by these programs. Additionally, these therapies may be most helpful when combined with other mind-body and educational therapies as a palatable option for improving movement capacity and autonomic dysfunction. One successful example is a pilot study of 28 subjects with FM who completed eight weeks of a program focused on education/cognitive-behavioral component, relaxation/meditation, and Qigong, which noted significant post-treatment and four-month follow-up improvement in the FIQ, tender points, and pain threshold (84).

DIET AND DIETARY SUPPLEMENTS

Elevated body mass index (BMI) has been linked to poorer outcomes in FM, including tenderness measures, quality of life, and physical functioning (78). Thus, on a very basic level, dietary management can be helpful as part of an approach to improving BMI and optimizing dietary and nutrient intake. Nutritional guidance and registered dietician consultation, if available, should be considered in all FM patients, especially those with elevated BMI.

In addition, dietary interventions and restriction have been advocated in FM as an approach to potentially decrease introduction of dietary allergens, excitotoxins, and proinflammatory compounds. Several small trials have noted benefit with use of a vegetarian, elimination, or partial fasting regimen (85,86). Because of the size of these trials, it is difficult to make any conclusion regarding the large-scale benefit of these types of diets. However, it is prudent in any FM patient, especially those with irritable bowel or other comorbidities, such as headache, which may have a dietary trigger, to set up consultation with a dietician to discuss appropriate meal planning to minimize potential triggers and ensure appropriate nutrient intake.

In addition to dietary interventions, a host of dietary supplements have been utilized in the setting of FM because of their potential benefit in the setting of nutritional deficiency, mitochondrial dysfunction, and/or neurotransmitter support. Unfortunately, very few of these agents have been tested in a rigorous manner and are more typically utilized in an empirical manner. A few of the more common supplements examined in the setting of FM are noted below.

Acetyl-L-Carnitine

Carnitine and, its more typical replacement form, acetyl-L-carnitine (LAC) are essential for energy production through their role as mitochondrial energy-transfer factors. In a multicenter study of 120 FM subjects, LAC was replaced at 1000 mg oral and 500 IM per day versus placebo for two weeks. This was followed by 1500 mg LAC or placebo per day for eight weeks. After six weeks, there were significant differences in pain, including tender points as well as depression and SF-36 scores in the active versus placebo group (87).

S-adenosyl-L-methionine

S-adenosyl-L-methionine (SAMe) has been thought to be helpful in FM due to its potential analgesic and serotonin upregulation roles. There is good support for its role as an antidepressant in studies versus placebo or other antidepressants at doses of 400 to 1600 mg/day orally where it is typically well tolerated (88). Two small trials using SAMe specifically in FM noted benefit in pain and related mood disturbance after use at 800 mg/day orally for six weeks (89,90). No significant benefit was noted with short-term (10 day) intravenously administered SAMe (91). Overall, because of the size of these trials, it is difficult to make any conclusions regarding this intervention specifically in FM. However, because of SAMe's benefit in the setting of depression, this may be a viable option for patients who have failed other treatments and may benefit from a minimum six-week trial of SAMe titrated to 800 mg/day. Caution is needed for patients with severe depression, bipolar disorder, or those taking other serotonergic agents.

Vitamin D

Several trials have noted deficient or suboptimal 25-hydroxyvitamin D levels in FM patients at higher than expected levels (92). Additionally, hypovitaminosis D in FM has been linked to worsening anxiety and depression (93). Recent research has also noted associations between hypovitaminosis D and increased cardio-vascular disease, several types of cancer, and all-cause mortality (94). Although there is no definitive evidence that replacement will improve FM symptoms, because of the negative health implications of hypovitaminosis D, clinicians should consider testing appropriate FM patients to detect and replete cases of depletion.

Other Biologicals
A number of other biologicals including serotonin precursors [5-HTP (5-hydroxytryptophan) (95,96) and melatonin (97)], magnesium (typically in combination with malic acid) (98), chlorella (99), topical capsaicin (100), and D-ribose (101) have demonstrated preliminary positive findings awaiting confirmation in larger well-controlled trials.

INTEGRATIVE/MULTIDISCIPLINARY CARE
A small number of studies have attempted to determine the benefit of integrative therapy on the outcome of FM. One of the better trials in this area (as mentioned earlier) was done by Rooks et al., who examined four interventions in 207 women with confirmed FM over 16 weeks (1). These interventions included exercise (either aerobic and flexibility or combined with strength training), education through the Arthritis Foundation based education program (FSCH), or a combination of education and exercise. These results showed minimal benefit with education alone, moderate benefit with exercise (aerobic with or without strength training), and most impressive benefit with combination of exercise with education assessed on the FM Impact Questionnaire and 36-Item Short-Form Health Survey. Most impressive was the fact that gains made with an integrative approach sustained at six months. The authors concluded that exercise, including simple walking, strength training, and strengthening, all improved functional status and that these gains were enhanced with education focused on targeted self-management.

In another integrative trial of 79 FM subjects, a six-week multidisciplinary rehabilitation program was compared to standard care (102). The multi-disciplinary group received 18 group exercise therapy sessions, 2 group pain and stress management lectures, 1 group education lecture, 1 group dietary lecture, and 2 massage therapy sessions. At trial completion the intervention group, in comparison to the control group, experienced statistically significant changes in average pain intensity, pain-related disability, self-perceived health status, and depressed mood. At 15 months these benefits were maintained versus standard care and additional reductions in medication (prescription and nonprescription) were noted. Finally, in Hadhazy et al.'s systematic review of MBTs for FM, the regimen that provided the greatest long-term benefit was MBTs combined with exercise (63).

CONCLUSION AND COORDINATION OF CARE
FM is a complex disorder that involves both central and peripheral sensitization causing pain amplification and multisystem dysfunction creating significant autonomic, musculoskeletal, and psychological sequelae. Because of the

sometimes-disparate presentation of patients with FM, it is imperative to individualize care. In addition, because of several factors including high levels of treatment failure, potential sensitivity to pharmacological interventions, and preference for specific treatment options, it is imperative for clinicians to be aware of NP/CAM options and to actively engage patient in discussion and coordination of these therapies when appropriate. Several table and figure resources are provided to enable initial and ongoing discussion and management of NP/CAM options in FM.

Several of the therapies reviewed in this chapter can provide safe, effective avenues of treatment for FM and its comorbidities. In many cases, the clinician is key in helping FM patients to practically incorporate the various NP/CAM options available to come up with a success integrative management plan. If properly coordinated, there is evidence that an integrative/multidisciplinary approach, which typically involves both MBT and exercise, may be more effective than monotherapy in creating a more function FM patient with self-management skills. In the future we look forward to addition research that helps to understand the synergy of NP/CAM therapies with conventional pharmacological care.

REFERENCES

1. Rooks DS, Gautam S, Romeling M, et al. Group exercise, education, and combination self-management in women with FM: a randomized trial. Arch Intern Med 2007; 167(20):2192–2200.
2. Wetzel MS, Eisenberg DM, Kaptchuk TJ. Courses involving complementary and alternative medicine at US medical schools. JAMA 1998; 280(9):784–787.
3. NIH Center for Complementary and Alternative Medicine (NCCAM). Available at: http://nccam.nih.gov/health/whatiscam/#sup2. Accessed October 23, 2006.
4. Wolsko PM, Eisenberg DM, Davis RB, et al. Patterns and perceptions of care for treatment of back and neck pain: results of a national survey. Spine 2003; 28(3): 292–297.
5. Barnes PM, Powell-Griner E, McFann K, et al. Complementary and alternative medicine use among adults: United States, 2002. Adv Data 2004; (343):1–19.
6. Lind BK, Lafferty WE, Tyree PT, et al. Use of complementary and alternative medicine providers by FM patients under insurance coverage. Arthritis Rheum 2007; 57(1):71–76.
7. Pioro-Boisset M, Esdaile JM, Fitzcharles MA. Alternative medicine use in FM syndrome. Arthritis Care Res 1996; 9(1):13–17.
8. Nicassio PM, Schuman C, Kim J. Psychosocial factors associated with complementary treatment use in FM. J Rheumatol 1997; 24(10):2008–2013.
9. Astin JA. Why patients use alternative medicine: results of a National Study. JAMA 1998; 279:1548–1553.
10. Furnham A, Bhagrath R. A comparison of health beliefs and behaviours of clients of orthodox and complementary medicine. Br J Clin Psychol 1993; 32:237–246.
11. Callahan LF, Freburger JK, Mielenz TJ, et al. Medical skepticism and the use of complementary and alternative health care providers by patients followed by rheumatologists. J Clin Rheumatol 2008; 14(3):143–147.
12. Astin, JA, Pelletier KR, Marie A, et al. Complementary and alternative medicine use among elderly persons: one-year analysis of a blue shield medicare supplement. J Gerontol A Biol Sci Med Sci 2000; 55(1):M4–M9.
13. Bennett RM, Jones J, Turk DC, et al. An internet survey of 2,596 people with FM. BMC Musculoskelet Disord 2007; 8:27.
14. Penrod JR, Bernatsky S, Adam V, et al. Health services costs and their determinants in women with FM. J Rheumatol 2004; 31(7):1391–1398.

15. Ashar BH, Rice TN, Sisson SD. Physicians' understanding of the regulation of dietary supplements. Arch Intern Med 2007; 167(9):966–969.
16. Kemper KJ, Gardiner P, Gobble J, et al. Expertise about herbs and dietary supplements among diverse health professionals. BMC Complement Altern Med 2006; 6:15.
17. Harris Interactive® Health Care News nationwide survey. Anti-aging medicine, vitamins, minerals and food supplements (completed October 2002). Available at: http://www.supplementquality.com/news/Harris_survey.html. Accessed August 28, 2008. Additional information available at: http://www.harrisinteractive.com.
18. Washington TA, Fanciullo GJ, Sorensen JA, et al. Quality of chronic pain websites. Pain Med 2008; 9(8):994–1000 [Epub March 11, 2008].
19. Bell RF. Food and pain: should we be more interested in what our patients eat? Pain 2007; 129(1–2):5–7.
20. Smith R. Let food be your medicine. BMJ 2004; 328 (doi:10.1136/bmj.328.7433.0-g).
21. Wold RS, Wayne SJ, Waters DL, et al. Behaviors underlying the use of nonvitamin nonmineral dietary supplements in a healthy elderly cohort. J Nutr Health Aging 2007; 11(1):3–7.
22. Azaz-Livshits T, Muszkat M, Levy M, et al. Use of complementary alternative medicine in patients admitted to internal medicine wards. Int J Clin Pharmacol Ther 2002; 40(12):539–547.
23. Adler SR, Fosket JR. Disclosing complementary and alternative medicine use in the medical encounter: a qualitative study in women with breast cancer. J Fam Pract 1999; 48(6):453–458.
24. Hansrud DD, Engle DD, Scheitel SM, et al. Underreporting the use of dietary supplements and nonprescription medication among patients undergoing a periodic health examination. Mayo Clin Proc 1999; 74:443–447.
25. Corbin-Winslow L, Shapiro H. Physicians want education about CAM to enhance communication with their patients. Arch Intern Med 2002; 162(10):1176–1181.
26. Bonakdar R, Guarneri E, Costello R. Herbal and dietary supplement in cardiovascular care: efficacy and incorporation into practice. In: Vogel J, Krucoff M, eds. Integrative Cardiology: Complementary and Alternative Medicine for the Heart. New York, U.S.A.: McGraw-Hill Professional, 2007:138.
27. Federal Drug Administration Press Release: FDA announces plans to prohibit sales of dietary supplements containing ephedra, Dec 30, 2003. Available at: http://www.fda.gov/oc/initiatives/ephedra/december2003/. Accessed May 1, 2004.
28. Federal Drug Administration Medwatch Press Release: 2002 Safety Alert—SPES, PC SPES, June 5, 2002. Available at: http://www.fda.gov/medwatch/SAFETY/2002/spes_press2.htm. Accessed May 1, 2004.
29. FDA Issues Dietary Supplements Final Rule. Available at: http://www.fda.gov/bbs/topics/NEWS/2007/NEW01657.html. Accessed June 22, 2007.
30. Sim J, Adams N. Systematic review of randomized controlled trials of non-pharmacological interventions for FM. Clin J Pain 2002; 18(5):324–336.
31. Staud R. Treatment of FM and its symptoms. Expert Opin Pharmacother 2007; 8(11): 1629–1642.
32. Goldenberg DL. Multidisciplinary modalities in the treatment of FM. J Clin Psychiatry 2008; 69(suppl 2):30–34.
33. Carville SF, Arendt-Nielsen S, Bliddal H, et al. EULAR (European League Against Rheumatism) evidence-based recommendations for the management of FM syndrome. Ann Rheum Dis 2008; 67(4):536–541.
34. Pariente J, White T, Frackowiak R, et al. Expectancy and belief modulate the neuronal substrates of pain treated by acupuncture. Neuroimage 2005; 25:1161–1167.
35. Sprott H, Franke S, Kluge H, et al. Pain treatment of FM by acupuncture. Rheumatol Int 1998; 18:35–36.
36. Berman BM, Swyers JP, Ezzo J. The evidence for acupuncture as a treatment for rheumatic conditions. Rheum Dis Clin North Am 2000; 26:103–115.
37. Deluze C, Bosia L, Zirbs A, et al. Electroacupuncture in FM: results of a controlled trial. BMJ 1992; 305:1249–1252.

38. Mayhew E, Ernst E. Acupuncture for FM—a systematic review of randomized clinical trials. Rheumatology (Oxford) 2007; 46(5):801–804 [Epub December 19, 2006].
39. Lundeberg T, Lund I. Are reviews based on sham acupuncture procedures in FM syndrome (FMS) valid? Acupunct Med 2007; 25(3):100–106.
40. Martin DP, Sletten CD, Williams BA, et al. Improvement in FM symptoms with acupuncture: results of a randomized controlled trial. Mayo Clin Proc 2006; 81(6): 749–757.
41. Jeschonneck M, Grohmann G, Hein G, et al. Abnormal microcirculation and temperature in skin above tender points in patients with FM. Rheumatology (Oxford) 2000; 39(8):917–921.
42. Morf S, Amann-Vesti B, Forster A, et al. Microcirculation abnormalities in patients with FM - measured by capillary microscopy and laser fluxmetry. Arthritis Res Ther 2005; 7(2):R209–R216 [Epub December 10, 2004].
43. Altan L, Bingöl U, Aykaç M, et al. Investigation of the effects of pool-based exercise on FM syndrome. Rheumatol Int 2004; 24(5):272–277.
44. Evcik D, Kizilay B, Gökçen E. The effects of balneotherapy on FM patients. Rheumatol Int 2002; 22(2):56–59.
45. Evcik D, Yigit I, Pusak H, et al. Effectiveness of aquatic therapy in the treatment of FM syndrome: a randomized controlled open study. Rheumatol Int 2008; 28(9):885–890.
46. McVeigh JG, McGaughey H, Hall M, et al. The effectiveness of hydrotherapy in the management of FM syndrome: a systematic review. Rheumatol Int 2008; 29(2): 119–130.
47. Gür A, Karakoc M, Nas K, et al. Effects of low power laser and low dose amitriptyline therapy on clinical symptoms and quality of life in FM: a single-blind, placebo-controlled trial. Rheumatol Int 2002; 22(5):188–193 [Epub July 6, 2002].
48. Gür A, Karakoç M, Nas K, et al. Efficacy of low power laser therapy in FM: a single-blind, placebo-controlled trial. Lasers Med Sci 2002; 17(1):57–61.
49. Matsutani LA, Marques AP, Ferreira EA, et al. Effectiveness of muscle stretching exercises with and without laser therapy at tender points for patients with FM. Clin Exp Rheumatol 2007; 25(3):410–415.
50. Bach GL, Clement DB. Efficacy of Farabloc as an analgesic in primary FM. Clin Rheumatol 2007; 26(3):405–410.
51. Alfano AP, Taylor AG, Foresman PA. Static magnetic fields for treatment of FM: a randomized controlled trial. J Altern Complement Med 2001; 7(1):53–64.
52. Shupak NM, McKay JC, Nielson WR, et al. Exposure to a specific pulsed low-frequency magnetic field: a double-blind placebo-controlled study of effects on pain ratings in rheumatoid arthritis and FM patients. Pain Res Manag 2006; 11(2):85–90.
53. Thomas AW, Graham K, Prato FS, et al. A randomized, double-blind, placebo-controlled clinical trial using a low-frequency magnetic field in the treatment of musculoskeletal chronic pain. Pain Res Manag 2007; 12(4):249–258.
54. Roizenblatt S, Fregni F, Gimenez R, et al. Site-specific effects of transcranial direct current stimulation on sleep and pain in FM: a randomized, sham-controlled study. Pain Pract 2007; 7(4):297–306.
55. Passard A, Attal N, Benadhira R, et al. Effects of unilateral repetitive transcranial magnetic stimulation of the motor cortex on chronic widespread pain in FM. Brain 2007; 130(pt 10):2661–2670.
56. Kaada B. [Treatment of FM by low-frequency transcutaneous nerve stimulation]. Tidsskr Nor Laegeforen 1989; 109(29):2992–2995.
57. McMakin CR, Gregory W, Phillips T. Cytokine changes with microcurrent treatment of FM associated with cervical spine trauma. J Bodywork Movement Ther 2005; 9:169–176.
58. Lichtbroun AS, Raicer MM, Smith RB. The treatment of FM with cranial electro-therapy stimulation. J Clin Rheumatol 2001; 7(2):72–78.
59. Field T, Diego M, Cullen C, et al. FM pain and substance P decrease and sleep improved after massage therapy. J Clin Rheumatol 2002; 8:72–76.
60. Sunshine W, Field T, Quintino O, et al. FM benefits from massage therapy and transcutaneous electrical stimulation. J Clin Rheumatol 1996; 2:18–22.

61. Brattberg G. Connective tissue massage in the treatment of FM. Eur J Pain 1999; 3:235–244.
62. Alnigenis M, Bradley JD, Wallick J, et al. Massage therapy in the management of FM: a pilot study. J Musculoskelet Pain 2001; 9:55–67.
63. Hadhazy VA, Ezzo J, Creamer P, et al. Mind-body therapies for the treatment of FM. A systematic review. J Rheumatol 2000; 27:2911–2918.
64. Lorig KR, Ritter PL, Laurent DD, et al. The internet-based arthritis self-management program: a one-year randomized trial for patients with arthritis or FM. Arthritis Rheum 2008; 59(7):1009–1017.
65. Singh BB, Berman BM, Creamer P. A pilot study of cognitive behavioral therapy in FM. Altern Ther Health Med 1998; 4:67–70.
66. Nielson WR, Walker C, Mccain GA. Cognitive behavioral treatment of FM syndrome: preliminary findings. J Rheumatol 1992; 19:98–103.
67. White KP, Nielson WR. Cognitive behavioral treatment of FM syndrome: a follow-up assessment. J Rheumatol 1995; 22:717–721.
68. Cohen H, Neumann L, Shore M, et al. Autonomic dysfunction in patients with FM: application of power spectral analysis of heart rate variability. Semin Arthritis Rheum 2000; 29(4):217–227.
69. Hassett AL, Radvanski DC, Vaschillo EG, et al. A pilot study of the efficacy of heart rate variability (HRV) biofeedback in patients with FM. Appl Psychophysiol Biofeedback 2007; 32(1):1–10 [Epub January 12, 2007].
70. Buckelew SP, Conway R, Parker J, et al. Biofeedback/relaxation training and exercise interventions for FM: a prospective trial. Arthritis Care Res 1998; 11(3):196–209.
71. Kabat-Zinn J, Massion AO, Kristeller J, et al. Effectiveness of a meditation-based stress reduction program in the treatment of anxiety disorders. Am J Psychiatry 1992; 149(7):936–943.
72. Kaplan KH, Goldenberg DL, Galvin-Nadeau M. The impact of a meditation-based stress reduction program on FM. Gen Hosp Psychiatry 1993; 15(5):284–289.
73. Sephton SE, Salmon P, Weissbecker I, et al. Mindfulness meditation alleviates depressive symptoms in women with FM: results of a randomized clinical trial. Arthritis Rheum 2007; 57(1):77–85.
74. Grossman P, Tiefenthaler-Gilmer U, Raysz A, et al. Mindfulness training as an intervention for FM: evidence of postintervention and 3-year follow-up benefits in well-being. Psychother Psychosom 2007; 76(4):226–233.
75. Menzies V, Taylor AG, Bourguignon C. Effects of guided imagery on outcomes of pain, functional status, and self-efficacy in persons diagnosed with FM. J Altern Complement Med 2006; 12(1):23–30.
76. Fors EA, Sexton H, Götestam KG. The effect of guided imagery and amitriptyline on daily FM pain: a prospective, randomized, controlled trial. J Psychiatr Res 2002; 36(3): 179–187.
77. Carrico DJ, Peters KM, Diokno AC. Guided imagery for women with interstitial cystitis: results of a prospective, randomized controlled pilot study. J Altern Complement Med 2008; 14(1):53–60.
78. Neumann L, Lerner E, Glazer Y, et al. A cross-sectional study of the relationship between body mass index and clinical characteristics, tenderness measures, quality of life, and physical functioning in FM patients. Clin Rheumatol 2008; 27(12): 1543–1547.
79. Taggart HM, Arslanian CL, Bae S, et al. Effects of T'ai Chi exercise on FM symptoms and health-related quality of life. Orthop Nurs 2003; 22(5):353–360.
80. Haak T, Scott B. The effect of Qigong on FM (FMS): a controlled randomized study. Disabil Rehabil 2008; 30(8):625–633.
81. da Silva GD, Lorenzi-Filho G, Lage LV. Effects of yoga and the addition of Tui Na in patients with FM. J Altern Complement Med 2007; 13(10):1107–1113.
82. Mannerkorpi K, Arndorw M. Efficacy and feasibility of a combination of body awareness therapy and qigong in patients with FM: a pilot study. J Rehabil Med 2004; 36(6):279–281.

83. Astin JA, Berman BM, Bausell B. The efficacy of mindfulness meditation plus Qigong movement therapy in the treatment of FM: a randomized controlled trial. J Rheumatol 2003; 30(10):2257–2262.

84. Creamer P, Singh BB, Hochberg MC, et al. Sustained improvement produced by nonpharmacologic intervention in FM: results of a pilot study. Arthritis Care Res 2000; 13(4):198–204.

85. Kaartinen K, Lammi K, Hypen M. Vegan diet alleviates FM symptoms. Scand J Rheumatol 2000; 29(5):308–313.

86. Smith JD, Terpening CM, Schmidt SO, et al. Relief of FM symptoms following discontinuation of dietary excitotoxins. Ann Pharmacother 2001; 35(6):702–706.

87. Rossini M, Di Munno O, Valentini G, et al. Double-blind, multicenter trial comparing acetyl l-carnitine with placebo in the treatment of FM patients. Clin Exp Rheumatol 2007; 25(2):182–188.

88. Delle Chiaie R, Pancheri P, Scapicchio P. Efficacy and tolerability of oral and intramuscular S-adenosyl-L-methionine 1,4-butanedisulfonate (SAMe) in the treatment of major depression: comparison with imipramine in 2 multicenter studies. Am J Clin Nutr 2002; 76(5):1172S–1176S.

89. Tavoni A, Vitali C, Bombardieri S, et al. Evaluation of S-adenosylmethionine in primary FM. A double-blind crossover study. Am J Med 1987; 83(5A):107–110.

90. Jacobsen S, Danneskiold-Samsøe B, Andersen RB. Oral S-adenosylmethionine in primary FM. Double-blind clinical evaluation. Scand J Rheumatol 1991; 20(4):294–302.

91. Volkmann H, Nørregaard J, Jacobsen S, et al. Double-blind, placebo-controlled cross-over study of intravenous S-adenosyl-L-methionine in patients with FM. Scand J Rheumatol 1997; 26(3):206–211.

92. Mouyis M, Ostor AJ, Crisp AJ, et al. Hypovitaminosis D among rheumatology outpatients in clinical practice. Rheumatology (Oxford) 2008; 47(9):1348–1351.

93. Armstrong DJ, Meenagh GK, Bickle I, et al. Vitamin D deficiency is associated with anxiety and depression in FM. Clin Rheumatol 2007; 26(4):551–554.

94. Melamed ML, Michos ED, Post W, et al. 25-hydroxyvitamin D levels and the risk of mortality in the general population. Arch Intern Med 2008; 168(15):1629–1637.

95. Caruso I, Sarzi Puttini P, Cazzola M, et al. Double-blind study of 5-hydroxy-tryptophan versus placebo in the treatment of primary FM syndrome. J Int Med Res 1990; 18:201–209.

96. Sarzi Puttini P, Caruso I. Primary FM syndrome and 5-hydroxy-L-tryptophan: a 90-day open study. J Int Med Res 1992; 20(2):182–189.

97. Citera G, Arias MA, Maldonado-Cocco JA, et al. The effect of melatonin in patients with FM: a pilot study. Clin Rheumatol 2000; 19(1):9–13.

98. Russell IJ, Michalek JE, Flechas JD, et al. Treatment of FM syndrome with Super Malic: a randomized, double blind, placebo controlled, crossover pilot study. J Rheumatol 1995; 22:953–958.

99. Merchant RE, Carmack CA, Wise CM. Nutritional supplementation with Chlorella pyrenoidosa for patients with FM syndrome: a pilot study. Phytother Res 2000; 14:167–173.

100. McCarty DJ, Csuka M, McCarthy G, et al. Treatment of pain due to FM with topical capsaicin: a pilot study. Semin Arthritis Rheum 1994; 23:41–47.

101. Teitelbaum JE, Johnson C, St Cyr J. The use of D-ribose in chronic fatigue syndrome and FM: a pilot study. J Altern Complement Med 2006; 12(9):857–862.

102. Lemstra M, Olszynski WP. The effectiveness of multidisciplinary rehabilitation in the treatment of FM: a randomized controlled trial. Clin J Pain 2005; 21(2):166–174.

4 The Pharmacological Treatment of Fibromyalgia

Lesley M. Arnold
Department of Psychiatry, Women's Health Research Program, University of Cincinnati College of Medicine, Cincinnati, Ohio, U.S.A.

INTRODUCTION

This chapter focuses on recent randomized, controlled studies of the pharmacological treatment of fibromyalgia. Clinical recommendations for the management of fibromyalgia using medications will be based on the available evidence from these trials. Tremendous progress has been made in the treatment of fibromyalgia, and it is likely that treatment options will continue to expand for patients with fibromyalgia.

The goal of fibromyalgia treatment is to develop an individualized approach that takes into account the severity of the patient's pain, the presence and severity of other symptoms, comorbidities, or stressors, and the degree of functional impairment. The treatment plan includes the identification and treatment of all pain sources that may be present in addition to fibromyalgia, such as peripheral pain generators (e.g., comorbid osteoarthritis or neuropathic pain) or visceral pain (e.g., comorbid irritable bowel syndrome). It is also important to address other symptoms or disorders that commonly occur in patients with fibromyalgia, such as fatigue, sleep disturbances and comorbid sleep disorders (e.g., sleep apnea), cognitive impairment, stiffness, and mood or anxiety disorders. Finally, the treatment should strive to improve the patient's function and global health status. In most cases the management of fibromyalgia involves both pharmacological and nonpharmacological treatments.

Most of the fibromyalgia clinical trials conducted recently and reviewed below identified patients using the American College of Rheumatology (ACR) criteria for fibromyalgia, which include chronic (at least 3 months duration) of widespread pain and pain on palpation of at least 11 out of 18 tender point sites (1). Because fibromyalgia is a chronic pain disorder, the clinical trials have focused on a measure of pain severity as the primary outcome. Some of the studies were designed to meet U.S. Food and Drug Administration (FDA) standards for approval of a medication treatment for fibromyalgia. In the early designs of these studies, a pain severity outcome measure and a patient global assessment of change score were included to meet criteria for improvement in pain associated with fibromyalgia. In addition, the FDA originally recommended that studies show improvement in three primary outcomes in order to obtain a claim of management of the syndrome of fibromyalgia: pain, a patient global assessment of change score, and a measure of function. Furthermore, the randomized, controlled trials were required to be at least six months in duration. After several studies were initiated using the above guidelines, the FDA changed its requirements and indicated that a positive trial need only show significant reduction in pain severity, compared with placebo, over the course of a three-month trial to receive approval for the management of fibromyalgia. This background about FDA guidelines for fibromyalgia trials provides an explanation for some of the trial designs of medications that have received FDA approval for the management of fibromyalgia (pregabalin, duloxetine, and milnacipran). For example, some of the trials are six months in duration as originally required by the FDA, but the primary outcome is at the three-month endpoint, meeting the most recent FDA recommendations for trial duration.

While pain continues to be the primary measure of efficacy in clinical trials of medications, most studies have also included a measure of function and patient global assessment of improvement. With the recognition that patients with fibromyalgia experience multiple symptom domains in addition to pain, the studies have also included several secondary outcomes to determine whether a particular medication might have efficacy in other symptoms domains in addition to pain. Table 1 summarizes common outcome measures used in recent pharmacological trials in fibromyalgia.

TABLE 1 Common Outcome Measures in Fibromyalgia Clinical Trials

Outcome	Measure (Ref)	Description
Clinical Domains		
Pain	Brief Pain Inventory (short form) (BPI) (2)	Self-report of average pain severity during the past 24 hours on an 11-point numeric scale from 0 (no pain) to 10 (pain as bad as you can imagine). Also severity of worst pain, least pain during the past 24 hours, pain right now, and pain interference from 0 (does not interfere) to 10 (completely interferes) with general activity, mood, walking ability, normal work, relations with other people, sleep, and enjoyment of life
	Daily pain diary (paper or electronic)	Visual analog scale 0 (no pain) to 100 (worst possible pain), or 11-point numeric scale 0 (no pain) to 10 (worst possible pain)
Fatigue	Multidimensional Fatigue Inventory (MFI) (3)	20-item, self-report instrument designed to collect data on the following dimensions: general fatigue, physical fatigue, mental fatigue, reduced motivation, and reduced activity
	Multidimensional Assessment of Fatigue (MAF) (4)	The Multidimensional Assessment of Fatigue (MAF) scale contains 16 items and measures four dimensions of fatigue: severity, distress, degree of interference in activities of daily living, and timing. 14 items contain numerical rating scales and two items have multiple-choice responses
Sleep	Medical Outcomes Study Sleep Scale (5)	12 items that assess key constructs of sleep and generates an overall sleep problems index
	Daily sleep diary (paper or electronic)	11-point numeric rating scale from 0 (best possible sleep) to 10 (worst possible sleep)
Mood	Hamilton Depression Rating Scale (HAM-D) (6)	17-item clinician-rated scale that measures multiple symptom domains of depression score range 0 (not at all depressed) to 52 (severely depressed)

(Continued)

TABLE 1   Common Outcome Measures in Fibromyalgia Clinical Trials (*Continued*)

Outcome	Measure (Ref)	Description
	Hospital Anxiety and Depression Scale (HADS) (7)	Self-report 14-item instrument that consists of two, 7-item subscales that measure the presence and severity of anxiety and depressive symptoms
Cognition	Multiple Ability Self-Report Questionnaire (MASQ) (8)	Self-report 38-item measure with items from five cognitive domains: language, visual-perceptual, verbal memory, visual memory, attention
Tenderness	Dolorimetry	Fischer dolorimeter (9) with rubber disc of 1 cm^2 applied to 18 tender point sites to determine pressure pain threshold and tender point count (number of tender points with a threshold of ≤ 4 kg/cm^2)
Function/quality of life	Fibromyalgia Impact Questionnaire (FIQ) (10)	20-item, self-administered questionnaire that measures multiple fibromyalgia symptoms and function domains over the past week
	Medical Outcomes Study Short Form 36 (SF-36) (11)	Patient-rated questionnaire that measures eight health concepts: physical functioning, role limitations due to physical problems, social functioning, bodily pain, mental health, role limitations due to emotional problems, vitality, general health perceptions. Physical component summary and mental component summary scales are based on the results of the eight scales
	Sheehan Disability Scale (12)	Self-report scale that rates impairment in work/school, social life, and family life/home responsibility on a 10-point scale
	Quality of Life in Depression Scale (13)	34-item, self-report questionnaire that assesses the impact of depressive symptoms on quality of life
	EuroQoL Questionnaire-5 Dimensions (14)	Self-report, generic health-related quality of life measure that assesses mobility, self-care, usual activities, pain/discomfort, and anxiety/depression
Global Assessment	Patient Global Impression of Improvement/Change (PGI-I or PGIC)	Self-report scale ranging from 1 (very much better) to 7 (very much worse)
	Clinical Global Impression of Severity (CGI-S) (15)	Clinician-rated scale ranging from 1 (normal, not at all ill) to 7 (among the most extremely ill patients)

PHARMACOLOGICAL TREATMENTS OF FIBROMYALGIA
Serotonin and Norepinephrine Reuptake Inhibitors

There is evidence that fibromyalgia is associated with aberrant central nervous system (CNS) processing of pain (16–19). Serotonergic and noradrenergic neurons are implicated in the mediation of endogenous pain inhibitory mechanisms through the descending inhibitory pain pathways in the brain and spinal cord (20–22). Dysfunction in serotonin and norepinephrine in these pain inhibitory pathways may contribute to the development of persistent pain associated with fibromyalgia and some other chronic pain conditions (23–27). Medications that inhibit the reuptake of serotonin and norepinephrine and thereby increase serotonin- and norepinephrine-mediated neurotransmission may correct a functional deficit of serotonin and norepinephrine in these descending inhibitory pain pathways and reduce pain. In both preclinical and clinical studies, it appears that medications with combined effects on serotonin and norepinephrine have more antinociceptive activity than those with effects on serotonin alone (28). Many medications that enhance serotonin and norepinephrine neurotransmission are also antidepressant or anxiolytic, but the antinociceptive activities of these medications are largely independent of their effects on mood, making them potentially efficacious for patients with or without depressive or anxiety symptoms (29).

Cyclic Medications

A meta-analysis (30) assessed nine placebo-controlled trials of cyclic drugs that inhibit the reuptake of both serotonin and norepinephrine, including the tricyclic antidepressants (TCAs) amitriptyline (31–34); dothiepin, which is structurally similar to amitriptyline and doxepin (35); cyclobenzaprine (32,36–38), which has structural and pharmacological properties of other TCAs (39); clomipramine (40); and the tetracyclic maprotiline (40). Seven outcome measures were assessed, including the patients' self-ratings of pain, stiffness, fatigue, and sleep; the patient and the physician global assessment of improvement; and the tender points. The largest effect was found in measures of sleep quality, with more modest changes in tender point measures and stiffness. Thus the most consistent improvement could be attributed to the sedative properties of these medications.

The results of another meta-analysis of randomized, placebo-controlled studies of cyclobenzaprine were consistent with the meta-analysis by Arnold et al. (2000) (30). Cyclobenzaprine treatment resulted in moderate improvement in sleep, modest improvement in pain, and no improvement in fatigue or tender points (41).

Although the meta-analyses indicate that the overall effect of cyclic drugs on most symptoms of fibromyalgia was moderate, possibly related to the low doses that were typically evaluated, TCAs continue to be recommended for the treatment of patients with fibromyalgia, usually as a nighttime medication (42). However, even at low doses (e.g., amitriptyline 25 mg/day), many patients experience problems with the safety and tolerability of these medications related to their anticholinergic, antiadrenergic, antihistaminergic, and quinidine-like effects (43).

Selective Serotonin and Norepinephrine Reuptake Inhibitors

Selective dual serotonin and norepinephrine reuptake inhibitors (SNRIs) act on the serotonin and norepinephrine reuptake transporters, but unlike the cyclic medications, do not interact with adrenergic, cholinergic, or histaminergic receptors, or sodium channels, and lack many of the side effects of cyclic medications.

Venlafaxine

Venlafaxine was the first newer-generation antidepressant to be classified as an SNRI. Venlafaxine sequentially engages serotonin uptake inhibition at low doses

(75 mg/day) and norepinephrine uptake inhibition at higher doses (375 mg/day), which is consistent with venlafaxine's ascending dose-antidepressant response curve (44). In a pilot, open-label study of venlafaxine in fibromyalgia, 15 patients were treated for eight weeks at a mean dose of 167 (SD ± 76) mg/day and reported significant improvement in pain, fatigue, sleep quality, feeling upon awakening, morning stiffness, depressive and anxiety symptoms, global assessment, and quality of life (45). By contrast, a six-week, randomized, placebo-controlled, double-blind trial of a fixed, low dose of venlafaxine (75 mg/day) in the treatment of fibromyalgia (46) found that venlafaxine, compared with placebo, did not significantly improve the primary measures of pain. The low dose of venlafaxine used in the controlled trial may explain the discrepant results, because venlafaxine at 75 mg/day may have selective serotonergic activity, which makes it less antinociceptive than higher doses of venlafaxine that may have dual activity on serotonin and norepinephrine. More trials of higher doses of venlafaxine (at least 150 mg/day or higher) are needed to determine the efficacy of venlafaxine in fibromyalgia.

Duloxetine
Duloxetine, a potent SNRI with dual reuptake inhibition of serotonin and norepinephrine over the entire clinically relevant dose range (47), is a safe, tolerable, and effective antidepressant (48–50) that also significantly reduces painful physical symptoms associated with major depressive disorder (51). In nondepressed patients with diabetes, duloxetine effectively reduces diabetic peripheral neuropathic pain (52,53), supporting an analgesic effect of duloxetine that is independent of its effects on mood. Duloxetine is currently indicated by the FDA for the acute and maintenance treatment of major depressive disorder in adults, acute treatment of generalized anxiety disorder in adults, the management of neuropathic pain associated with diabetic peripheral neuropathy in adults. In June 2008, duloxetine became the first SNRI to be approved by the FDA for the management of fibromyalgia in adults (54). Table 2 summarizes randomized, controlled trials of duloxetine in fibromyalgia. The data from the two published pivotal trials will be presented in detail below.

The first pivotal trial, a randomized, placebo-controlled, double-blind, parallel-group, multisite, 12-week study of duloxetine monotherapy in fibromyalgia, tested the safety and efficacy of both 60 mg twice a day (BID) and 60 mg once a day (QD) in 354 women with fibromyalgia with or without current major depressive disorder (56). The primary outcome measure was pain severity as measured by the self-reported Brief Pain Inventory (short form) average pain severity score (2). Compared to placebo, duloxetine 60 mg QD and duloxetine 60 mg BID resulted in significantly greater improvement in the Brief Pain Inventory pain severity and interference scores, and other secondary outcomes including the total score of the Fibromyalgia Impact Questionnaire (10), the Clinical Global Impression of Severity, and the Patient Global Impression of Improvement (15). Several quality of life measures significantly improved in both duloxetine groups compared to the placebo group including the Quality of Life in Depression Scale (13) total score, the Sheehan Disability Scale (12) total score, and the Medical Outcomes Study Short Form 36 (SF-36) (11) mental subscore, bodily pain, mental health, role limit emotional, role limit physical, and vitality. There were no significant differences between duloxetine 60 mg QD

TABLE 2 Randomized, Double-Blind, Placebo-Controlled Fibromyalgia Trials of Selective SNRIs

SNRI study	SNRI (dosage, mg/day)	Study design (no. of patients)	Duration (wk)	Significant efficacy outcomes, treatment vs. placebo
Duloxetine				
Arnold et al. (2004) (55)	Duloxetine (120)	Duloxetine vs. placebo, parallel (207)	12	*Primary measure:* FIQ total score (FIQ pain score improved in women only) *Secondary measures:* FIQ stiffness scores; BPI pain severity and interference from pain; tender points; CGI-S; PGI-I; QLDS; SDS; SF-36 physical subscore and bodily pain, general health perception, mental health, physical function, vitality scores
Arnold et al. (2005) (56)	Duloxetine (60 and 120)	Duloxetine vs. placebo, parallel (354)	12	*Primary measure:* BPI average pain severity *Secondary measures:* BPI interference from pain; FIQ total score; tender points (120 mg only); CGI-S; PGI-I; QLDS; SDS; SF-36 mental subscore and scores for social function (60 mg only), physical function (120 mg only), bodily pain, mental health, role limit emotional and physical, and vitality
Russell et al. (2008) (57)	Duloxetine (20, 60, 120)	Duloxetine vs. placebo, parallel (520)	15 (primary endpoint), 28 (secondary endpoint)	*Primary measures at 15 wk:* BPI average pain severity (60 mg, 120 mg); PGI-I *Primary measures at 28 wk:* BPI average pain severity; PGI-I (20 mg, 120 mg) *Secondary measures at 15 wk:* FIQ total score; MFI reduced motivation (60 mg, 120 mg); MFI mental fatigue (60 mg only); MFI reduced activity (20 mg, 120 mg); CGI-S (60 mg, 120 mg); SF-36 mental component summary (60 mg, 120 mg); EQ-5D (20 mg only) *Secondary measures at 28 wk:* MFI mental fatigue; MFI physical fatigue (120 mg only); MFI reduced motivation (120 mg only); MFI reduced activity (120 mg only); CGI-S; SF-36 mental component summary (120 mg only); EQ-5D (20 mg only)

(Continued)

TABLE 2 Randomized, Double-Blind, Placebo-Controlled Fibromyalgia Trials of Selective SNRIs (*Continued*)

SNRI study	SNRI (dosage, mg/day)	Study design (no. of patients)	Duration (wk)	Significant efficacy outcomes, treatment vs. placebo
Milnacipran				
Gendreau et al. (2005) (58)	Milnacipran (up to 200)	Milnacipran vs. placebo, parallel (125)	12	*Secondary measures*: pain (weekly e-diary pain score, paper daily and weekly scores, present pain score), PGIC; FIQ physical function, days felt good, pain, fatigue, and morning stiffness scores
Mease et al. (2008) (59)	Milnacipran (100, 200)	Milnacipran vs. placebo, parallel (888)	15 (primary endpoint), 27 (secondary endpoint)	*Primary measure at 15 wk*: fibromyalgia composite responder; pain composite responder (200 mg only) *Primary measure at 27 wk*: pain composite responder (200 mg only) *Secondary measures at 15 wk*: weekly average of 24-hour pain scores and real-time pain scores, and weekly pain scores (200 mg only); SF-36 physical functioning (200 mg only), bodily pain (200 mg only), and mental health (200 mg only); MFI total score; MASQ (200 mg only) *Secondary measures at 27 wk*: weekly average of 24-hour pain scores and real-time pain scores (200 mg only); SF-36 bodily pain and mental health; MFI total score (200 mg only); MASQ (200 mg only)

Abbreviations: SNRI, serotonin and norepinephrine reuptake inhibitors; FIQ, Fibromyalgia Impact Questionnaire; PGIC, Patient Global Impression of Change; BPI, Brief Pain Inventory; CGI-S, clinician global impression of severity; PGI-I, patient global impression of improvement; QLDS, Quality of Life in Depression Scale; SDS, Sheehan Disability Scale; SF-36, Medical Outcomes Study Short Form; MFI, Multidimensional Fatigue Inventory; EQ-5D, EuroQoL Questionnaire-5 dimensions; MASQ, Multiple Ability Self-Report Questionnaire.

and duloxetine 60 mg BID treatment groups in efficacy outcomes. However, only the duloxetine 60 mg BID dose, compared to placebo, significantly improved the tender point number and mean tender point pain thresholds that were assessed using a Fischer dolorimeter (9) applied to the 18 tender point sites defined by the ACR criteria (1). This suggests that a higher dose may be necessary to improve pressure pain thresholds, which have been found to be less responsive to treatment in previous fibromyalgia trials using tricyclics (30). In this trial, 26% of the patients had current major depressive disorder. Notably the treatment effect of duloxetine on pain reduction was independent of the effect on mood and the presence of major depressive disorder.

The most frequent side effect in patients in the duloxetine 60 mg QD and 60 mg BID groups was nausea, and the side effects were mild to moderate in severity for most patients. There were no clinically relevant differences between treatment groups in laboratory assessments, vital signs, or physical findings. Significantly more patients in the duloxetine 60 mg BID group than the placebo group discontinued treatment due to adverse events. This finding differs from the proof of concept duloxetine trial of 60 mg BID in which there were no differences between treatment groups in discontinuation due to treatment-emergent adverse events (55). This suggests that some patients would benefit from a lower duloxetine starting dose and slower titration. Indeed, the FDA prescribing information notes that some patients may benefit from starting at 30 mg QD for about a week to allow patients to adjust to the medication before increasing the dose. Although the pivotal trials of duloxetine in fibromyalgia included the 120 mg QD dose, the FDA-recommended dose for fibromyalgia is 60 mg QD. Nonetheless, some patients may have a better response at higher doses, either 90 mg QD (which has not yet been studied in fibromyalgia) or 120 mg QD.

The second pivotal trial, a randomized, placebo-controlled, double-blind, parallel-group, multisite, six-month study of duloxetine monotherapy in fibromyalgia, tested the safety and efficacy of 20 mg QD (after 3 months, the 20 mg QD group titrated to 60 mg QD), 60 mg QD, and 120 mg QD in 520 fibromyalgia patients (women and men) with or without current major depressive disorder (57). Compared to placebo-treated patients, patients treated with duloxetine 120 mg QD improved significantly more on the coprimary measures at three months and at the secondary endpoint of six months. Compared to placebo, treatment with duloxetine 60 mg QD also significantly improved the coprimary measures at three months and the Brief Pain Inventory score at six months. The 20 mg QD group did not experience significant improvement in pain at three months compared to placebo, but did have a significant improvement on the Patient Global Impressions of Improvement. At six months, significantly more patients treated with duloxetine 120 mg QD (36%), duloxetine 60 mg QD (33%), and the group of duloxetine-treated patients who were titrated from 20 to 60 mg QD in the last three months of the study (20/60 mg QD) (36%) compared with placebo (22%) had a 50% or more reduction in the Brief Pain Inventory average pain severity score. Response rates defined by 30% or more reduction in the pain score were significantly higher at six months only for the 20/60 mg QD group (52%) compared to placebo (37%). For secondary measures at the three-month endpoint, both duloxetine 120 mg QD and 60 mg QD had significantly greater improvement compared to placebo-treated patients in the Clinical Global Impression of Severity, Fibromyalgia Impact Questionnaire total score, SF-36 mental component score, and reduced motivation domain of the Multidimensional Fatigue Inventory measure (3). In this trial, 24% of the patients had current major depressive disorder. As in the other trials of duloxetine in fibromyalgia, the treatment effect of duloxetine on pain reduction was independent of the effect on mood and the presence of major depressive disorder.

The safety and tolerability findings in this study were consistent with the previous fibromyalgia pivotal trial, other duloxetine fibromyalgia studies, and findings in other patient populations. The most commonly reported treatment-emergent adverse events in placebo-controlled fibromyalgia studies that were reported at a rate of 5% or more and at least twice the rate of placebo were nausea, dry mouth, constipation, somnolence, decreased appetite, increased sweating, and agitation (54). A pooled analysis of almost 24,000 duloxetine patients from 64 studies found that the majority of the most commonly reported adverse effects occurred early in treatment and were mild to moderate in severity (60). In addition, an analysis of eight pooled double-blind studies demonstrated that nausea, the most frequently reported side effect, occurred in the first few weeks of treatment with duloxetine, and resolved for most patients within a few days to a week (61). Furthermore, an evaluation of over 8500 duloxetine-treated patients from 42 placebo-controlled studies found no increased cardiovascular risk associated with duloxetine (62).

Summary. The results of randomized, controlled trials of duloxetine in fibromyalgia demonstrate that duloxetine monotherapy at doses of 60 mg QD and 120 mg QD reduces pain and improves other key symptoms of fibromyalgia, such as mental fatigue, and is associated with improvement in function, health-related quality of life, and global assessments. Notably, duloxetine is efficacious in fibromyalgia patients with or without current depression, and the effect of duloxetine on reduction in pain appears to be independent of its effect on mood.

Milnacipran

Milnacipran is another SNRI that has been approved for treatment of depression since 1997 in parts of Europe, Asia, and elsewhere. In the United States, milnacipran has been studied for the treatment of fibromyalgia and has received FDA's approval for management of fibromyalgia in early 2009. Milnacipran is a dual serotonin and norepinephrine reuptake inhibition within its therapeutic dose range and also exerts mild N-methyl-D-aspartate (NMDA) inhibition (63). Like duloxetine and venlafaxine, milnacipran lacks the side effects of TCAs associated with antagonism of adrenergic, cholinergic, and histaminergic receptors. The proof of concept study in fibromyalgia as well as one of the pivotal trials will be reviewed here. Table 2 summarizes the results of these studies.

The proof of concept study was a double-blind, placebo-controlled, multicenter trial of 125 patients (98% women) with fibromyalgia who were randomized to receive placebo or milnacipran for four weeks of dose escalation to the maximally tolerated dose followed by eight weeks of stable dose (25–200 mg/day) (58). The study evaluated the efficacy and safety of two different dosing regimens of milnacipran monotherapy (once daily versus twice daily) for the treatment of fibromyalgia. The primary outcome measure was based on change in pain recorded on an electronic diary, comparing baseline to endpoint (last two weeks on treatment). The majority of milnacipran-treated patients titrated to the highest daily dose (200 mg), suggesting that milnacipran was well tolerated. Similar to the other drugs in this class, the most frequently reported adverse event was nausea, and most adverse events were mild to moderate and transient.

Patients treated with milnacipran on a twice-daily schedule experienced significant improvement in pain compared to those on placebo. Significantly more patients receiving milnacipran twice daily (37%) reported a reduction in the weekly average pain scores by 50% or more, compared with 14% of patients in the placebo group. Milnacipran-treated patients on the once-daily schedule did not exhibit the same degree of improvement in pain, suggesting that dosing frequency is important in the use of milnacipran for pain associated with fibromyalgia. Both milnacipran groups (once-daily and twice-daily dosing) had significantly greater improvement on secondary measures, including the Patient Global Impression of Change score, and the physical function and "days felt good" subscales of the Fibromyalgia Impact Questionnaire. As in the duloxetine trials, patients were evaluated for psychiatric comorbidity and those with and without current major depressive disorder were included. Unlike the results of the duloxetine trials in which both depressed and nondepressed patients responded similarly to duloxetine, statistically greater improvement in pain reduction was seen in nondepressed patients versus depressed patients treated with milnacipran. The positive response in nondepressed patients suggests that, like duloxetine, the pain-relieving effects of milnacipran do not occur only through improvement in mood.

The first pivotal trial, a randomized, placebo-controlled, double-blind, parallel-group, multisite, 27-week study of milnacipran monotherapy in fibromyalgia, tested the safety and efficacy of 50 mg BID and 100 mg BID in 888 fibromyalgia patients (women and men) (59). Unlike the proof of concept study and the duloxetine clinical trials, patients with current major depressive disorder were excluded from the pivotal trial of milnacipran. Two composite responder definitions were used to classify each patient's individual response to therapy. The primary efficacy measure for fibromyalgia treatment was defined as the percentage of patients who, at weeks 15 and 27, concurrently met all of the following three criteria: (*i*) 30% or more pain improvement as assessed by the change from baseline in 24-hour morning recall pain collected from daily electronic diaries and averaged for the 14 days immediately preceding and including study visit days, (*ii*) a rating of "very much improved" or "much improved" on the Patient Global Impression of Change score, and (*iii*) 6 or more point improvement from baseline in physical function as measured by the SF-36 physical component score. The primary efficacy measure for treatment of pain of fibromyalgia was defined as the pain improvement and Patient Global Impression of Change thresholds indicated above. Compared to placebo-treated patients, a significantly higher percentage of patients treated with milnacipran 50 mg BID and 100 mg BID met the criteria as fibromyalgia composite responders at 15 weeks, but not at 27 weeks. Significantly more patients on 100 mg BID of milnacipran, but not milnacipran 50 mg BID, met criteria as composite responders for pain of fibromyalgia at 15 weeks and 27 weeks, as compared to patients on placebo. At 15 weeks, patients on milnacipran 100 mg BID had significantly greater improvement compared to placebo on the SF-36 domains of physical functioning, bodily pain, and mental health. At 27 weeks, the 100 mg BID dose of milnacipran, compared to placebo, significantly improved the weekly averages of 24-hour recall and real-time pain scores. At 27 weeks, both doses of milnacipran showed improvement in the SF-36 domains of bodily pain and mental health. Treatment with milnacipran 100 mg BID, compared to placebo, significantly reduced fatigue at weeks 15 and 27, as measured by the Multidimensional Fatigue Inventory, particularly the reduced motivation domain. Changes in the Multiple Ability Self-Report Questionnaire (8), which assesses difference in the patients' perception of their cognitive function, were significantly improved for patients on milnacipran 100 mg BID compared to placebo-treated patients at 15 and 27 weeks.

Most treatment-emergent adverse events were mild to moderate in severity. Adverse events occurring in at least 5% of patients in either milnacipran treatment group and at an incidence of at least two times that of placebo patients included constipation, increased sweating, hot flush, vomiting, heart rate increase, dry mouth, palpitations, and hypertension. The most common adverse event in all treatment groups was nausea, which tended to be dose related, mild to moderate in severity, and typically resolved in two to four weeks with continued therapy. A small percentage of milnacipran-treated patients (<2%) had a potentially clinically significant rise in supine heart rate relative to the placebo group. Mean change in blood pressure and heart rate as well as potentially clinically significant change or sustained increase in vital signs were similar in milnacipran- and placebo-treated patients.

Summary. The results of randomized, controlled trials of milnacipran in fibromyalgia demonstrate that milnacipran monotherapy at doses of 50 mg BID and 100 mg BID reduces pain and improves global assessments, function, and quality of life as well as other key symptoms of fibromyalgia, such as fatigue and cognition.

Selective Serotonin Reuptake Inhibitors
Selective serotonin reuptake inhibitors (SSRIs) that have a high affinity for the serotonin transporter have been evaluated in six double-blind, placebo-controlled trials in fibromyalgia: two with citalopram (64,65), three with fluoxetine (34,66,67), and one with paroxetine CR (68). The results for SSRIs are mixed, suggesting that medications with selective serotonin effects are less consistent in relieving pain and other symptoms associated with fibromyalgia. Indeed, there is evidence that serotonin has pro- and antinociceptive actions in the descending pain modulatory pathways in the brain and spinal cord (22). Therefore, while there may be a synergistic effect of serotonin and norepinephrine that mediates the antinociceptive effects of the SNRIs, medications that effect only serotonin may be more weakly antinociceptive (28).

Citalopram
In the first study of citalopram in fibromyalgia in which 42 patients with fibromyalgia were randomized to citalopram (20–40 mg/day) or placebo for eight weeks, there were no significant differences in efficacy between the citalopram and placebo groups (64). In the second randomized, double-blind, placebo-controlled, four-month study of 40 women with fibromyalgia, citalopram (20–40 mg/day) significantly decreased depressive symptoms compared with placebo, but there were no significant differences between groups in other symptoms of fibromyalgia (65). Therefore, citalopram, which has the highest selectivity for the serotonin reuptake transporters among the SSRIs, was not effective for the treatment of fibromyalgia in two controlled, albeit small, studies.

Fluoxetine

The first fluoxetine trial of 20 mg/day did not find a significant therapeutic effect over placebo (66). In two other controlled trials, fluoxetine was superior to placebo in reducing pain and other symptoms associated with fibromyalgia (34,67). In a double-blind, crossover study in which 19 subjects with fibromyalgia received four six-week trials of fluoxetine 20 mg/day, amitriptyline 25 mg/day, their combination, or placebo, both fluoxetine and amitriptyline produced significant improvement in pain, global well-being and function compared with placebo. Combination treatment produced significantly greater improvement than either drug did alone (34). In a randomized, placebo-controlled, parallel-group, flexible-dose, 12-week trial of fluoxetine in fibromyalgia, 60 female patients who did not have any current comorbid psychiatric disorders or depressive symptoms were randomized to receive fluoxetine 10 to 80 mg/day or placebo and were evaluated with the Fibromyalgia Impact Questionnaire total and pain scores as the primary outcome measures (67). Patients receiving fluoxetine (mean dose 45 ± 25 mg/day) had significantly greater reductions in Fibromyalgia Impact Questionnaire total and pain scores compared to the placebo group. As was seen in the duloxetine trials, the effect of fluoxetine on reduction of pain associated with fibromyalgia appeared to be independent of an effect on mood. Fluoxetine was generally well tolerated; there were no significant differences between the two groups in dropouts due to side effects. Because of the beneficial effects of higher doses of fluoxetine in this study, some patients who fail to respond to a 20 mg/day dose of fluoxetine may improve with higher doses, if tolerated. The positive studies of fluoxetine suggest that this SSRI might have unique pharmacological properties that may underlie its efficacy in fibromyalgia. Fluoxetine has been shown to increase extracellular concentrations of norepinephrine as well as serotonin in the prefrontal cortex in preclinical models (69). Consistent with the results of antidepressants that have dual effects on serotonin and norepinephrine, SSRIs that have additional effects on norepinephrine, at adequate doses, may also be effective for fibromyalgia.

Paroxetine

A randomized, double-blind, placebo-controlled, flexible-dose, 12-week trial of paroxetine CR (dose 12.5–62.5 mg/day) in 116 patients with fibromyalgia defined response to treatment as 25% or more reduction in the Fibromyalgia Impact Questionnaire total score (68). Significantly more patients in the paroxetine CR group (57%) responded compared to placebo (33%). However, there were no significant differences between treatment groups in the reduction of pain. Like fluoxetine, paroxetine at higher doses may exhibit norepinephrine transporter inhibition (70), but more study of this SSRI is needed in fibromyalgia to establish whether, at higher doses, there is a consistent effect on pain.

Selective Norepinephrine Reuptake Inhibitors

Norepinephrine is believed to have predominantly pain inhibitory activity in the descending pain modulatory pathways in the brain and spinal cord (22), and the antinociceptive effects of norepinephrine reuptake inhibitors (NRIs) have been demonstrated in preclinical models of pain (28). Esreboxetine, a highly selective NRI that is not yet available in the United States, is the active enantiomer in racemic reboxetine, which is currently marketed in over 40 countries outside the United States as an antidepressant.

The proof of concept study of esreboxetine in fibromyalgia was a randomized, double-blind, placebo-controlled, parallel-group, multicenter, eight-week study of esreboxetine monotherapy in fibromyalgia that evaluated the safety and efficacy of 2 mg QD to 8 mg QD in 515 women and men with fibromyalgia (71). Compared to the placebo group, the esreboxetine-treated patients experienced significantly greater improvement in the mean pain score at endpoint. Significantly more patients treated with esreboxetine QD (38%) compared with placebo (23%) had a 30% or more reduction in the mean pain score. In addition, significantly more patients in the esreboxetine-treated patients (18%) compared to placebo (8%) had a 50% or more reduction in the mean pain score. Compared with placebo, esreboxetine resulted in significantly greater improvement in secondary outcomes, including the total score of the Fibromyalgia Impact Questionnaire, the Patient Global Impression of Change score, and the Multidimensional Assessment of Fatigue (4).

The side effects that were reported more frequently in patients in the esreboxetine group were constipation, insomnia, dry mouth, headache, nausea, dizziness, and increased sweating. The majority of adverse events reported were mild to moderate in severity. There were no clinically relevant differences between treatment groups in laboratory assessments, vital signs, or physical findings. There was a median increase in sitting pulse rate of 7 beats/min in the esreboxetine group at the end of the study. However, there were no accompanying symptomatic adverse events or corresponding changes in systolic or diastolic blood pressure.

Dopamine Agonists
Pramipexole
Excessive adrenergic arousal may fragment sleep, and enhancement of dopaminergic neurotransmission at the dopamine-3 receptors in the mesolimbic hippocampus may reduce expression of arousal and improve sleep. In addition, mesolimbic, mesocortical, and nigrostriatal dopamine pathways are involved in the inhibition of nociception, primarily the affective component. Dopamine may also be involved in the modulation of descending control, although the precise mechanism remains to be elucidated (22). Pramipexole, a dopamine-3 receptor agonist, was added on to existing pharmacological and nonpharmacological therapies in patients with fibromyalgia in a 14-week, single-center, randomized, placebo-controlled study (72).

Compared with the placebo group, those patients receiving pramipexole titrated over 12 weeks to 4.5 mg every evening had significant improvement in pain, fatigue, function, and global status. A gradual titration of pramipexole was well tolerated; weight loss and increased anxiety were significantly more common in patients on pramipexole. Sleep was not assessed in the study, despite the proposed role of dopamine-3 receptor agonists in reducing adrenergic arousal in patients with fibromyalgia. The study was also difficult to interpret because the participants were taking concomitant medications (about half on narcotic analgesics) for fibromyalgia. More studies of dopamine agonists are needed to understand their potential role in the treatment of patients with fibromyalgia.

Alpha-2-Delta Ligands
In addition to the possible role of dysfunction in the descending pain inhibitory pathways in fibromyalgia, there is also emerging evidence of the involvement of other central pain mechanisms in fibromyalgia, including central pain sensitization.

In central pain sensitization, there is an amplification of nociceptive impulses that is a result of the plasticity of neuronal synapses following past pain experiences (73). Input from nociceptive afferent nerves causes a release of excitatory neurotransmitters such as glutamate and substance P in the dorsal horn of the spinal cord, which may contribute to neuronal hyperactivity and central sensitization.

Pregabalin and gabapentin are alpha-2-delta (α2-δ) ligands that have analgesic, anxiolytic, and anticonvulsant activities. The analgesic action of both drugs is thought to be mediated through the α2-δ protein, an auxiliary subunit of voltage-dependent calcium channels. By binding to α2-δ subunits and modulating the influx of calcium ions into hyperexcited neurons, pregabalin and gabapentin reduce the synaptic release of several neurotransmitters believed to play a role in pain processing, including glutamate and substance P. This reduction in synaptic activity may account for the reduction in neuronal excitability and ultimately the analgesic action of these medications (74–76).

Pregabalin

Pregabalin is approved by the FDA for neuropathic pain associated with diabetic peripheral neuropathy, postherpetic neuralgia, adjunctive therapy for adults with partial onset seizures, and the management of fibromyalgia (77). Pregabalin was the first medication to be approved by the FDA for the management of fibromyalgia in adults. Table 3 summarizes the randomized, controlled trials of pregabalin in fibromyalgia. The data from the two published pivotal trials will be presented in detail below.

The first pivotal study of pregabalin in fibromyalgia was a multicenter, randomized, double-blind, placebo-controlled trial in which 750 (95% female) patients with fibromyalgia were randomized to pregabalin 150 mg BID, 225 mg BID, 300 mg BID, or placebo, for 14 weeks, following one week of single-blind administration of placebo (80). The primary efficacy outcome was comparison of endpoint mean pain scores, derived from daily diary ratings of pain intensity on a scale of 0 (no pain) to 10 (worst possible pain) between each of the pregabalin groups and the placebo group. If positive, additional primary efficacy parameters included the Patient Global Impression of Change and the Fibromyalgia Impact Questionnaire total score. Compared with placebo-treated patients, mean changes in pain scores at endpoint in all pregabalin-treated groups were significantly greater. In addition, compared with placebo, significantly more pregabalin-treated patients reported improvement on the Patient Global Impression of Change and, for the 225 mg BID and the 300 mg BID doses, significant improvements in total Fibromyalgia Impact Questionnaire score. Secondary outcomes that improved significantly in the pregabalin groups compared with placebo included the Medical Outcomes Study Sleep Problems Index (5) and the daily sleep-quality diary. Fatigue, as measured by the Multidimensional Assessment of Fatigue, did not improve significantly with pregabalin compared with placebo, but pregabalin 225 mg BID and 300 mg BID significantly improved the vitality score on the SF-36 compared with placebo. A significantly larger proportion of patients receiving pregabalin 150 mg BID (42%), 225 mg BID (50%), and 300 mg BID (48%) experienced a 30% or more reduction in the pain (diary) score compared with the placebo group (30%). Most adverse events were mild to moderate in severity and tended to be dose related. Dizziness and somnolence were the most common adverse events associated with pregabalin treatment. Other events reported by at least 5% of

TABLE 3 Randomized, Double-Blind, Placebo-Controlled Fibromyalgia Trials of α2-δ Ligands

α2-δ Study	α2-δ ligand (dosage, mg/day)	Study design (no. of patients)	Duration (wk)	Significant efficacy outcomes, treatment vs. placebo
Pregabalin				
Crofford et al. (2005) (78)	Pregabalin (150, 300, and 450)	Pregabalin vs. placebo, parallel (529)	8	*Primary measure:* mean daily pain score (daily diaries) (450 mg only) *Secondary measures:* sleep quality diary (300 mg, 450 mg); MOS sleep problem index; MAF global fatigue (300 mg, 450 mg); patient and clinician global impression of change (300 mg, 450 mg); SF-36 general health (150 mg, 300 mg, 450 mg), vitality (450 mg), bodily pain (450mg), social functioning (450 mg)
Mease et al. (2008) (79)	Pregabalin (300, 450, 600)	Pregabalin vs. placebo, parallel (748)	13	*Primary measures:* mean daily pain score (daily diaries); PGIC *Secondary measures:* sleep quality diary; MOS sleep problem index
Arnold et al. (2008) (80)	Pregabalin 300, 450, 600	Pregabalin vs. placebo, parallel (750)	14	*Primary measures:* mean daily pain score (daily diaries); PGIC; FIQ total (450 mg, 600 mg) *Secondary measures:* sleep quality diary; MOS sleep problem index; HADS anxiety score (600 mg only); SF-36 vitality (450 mg, 600 mg); SF-36 social functioning (450 mg only); SF-36 mental health (600 mg only), mental component score (600 mg only)
Crofford et al. (2008) (81)	Pregabalin 300, 450, 600	Open label phase to identify pregabalin responders, followed by randomization to placebo or pregabalin (1051)	6-wk open label, 26-wk double-blind phase	*Primary measure:* time to LTR on pain (or clinical worsening) significantly longer for pregabalin group than for patients on placebo *Secondary measures:* time to LTR significantly longer for pregabalin group than placebo patients on PGIC; FIQ total score; MOS sleep problem index; MAF; SF-36 physical and mental component scores
Gabapentin				
Arnold et al. (2007) (82)	Gabapentin (1200–2400)	Gabapentin vs. placebo, parallel (150)	12	*Primary measure:* BPI average pain severity *Secondary measures:* BPI interference from pain; FIQ total score; PGI-I; MOS sleep problem index; SF-36 vitality

Abbreviations: MOS, Medical Outcomes Study; MAF, Multidimensional Assessment of Fatigue; SF-36, Medical Outcomes Study Short Form; BPI, Brief Pain Inventory; PGI-I, patient global impression of improvement; PGIC, Patient Global Impression of Change; FIQ, Fibromyalgia Impact Questionnaire; HADS, Hospital Anxiety and Depression Scale; LTR, loss of therapeutic response.

patients in any of the treatment groups and more common in the combined pregabalin groups included increased weight, peripheral edema, fatigue, blurred vision, constipation, disturbance in attention, balance disorder, euphoric mood, sinusitis, back pain, dry mouth, increased appetite, and memory impairment. As recommended in the FDA prescribing information for pregabalin in fibromyalgia, all pregabalin-treated patients were started at 75 mg BID and titrated every three to four days; all patients received 150 mg BID by the end of the first week. Patients in the 225 mg BID and 300 mg BID groups continued escalating to their randomized dose by the end of week 2. Although not recommended in the FDA prescribing information, a lower starting dose (e.g., 75 mg QHS) and slower escalation to higher dosages, with most or all of the doses at bedtime, may decrease the incidence or severity of adverse events. Although the pivotal trials of pregabalin included a 300 mg BID dose, the FDA maximum recommended dose for fibromyalgia is 225 mg BID. However, some patients may respond better at the 300 mg BID dose.

The second pregabalin pivotal trial was a six-month study that assessed the durability of the effect of pregabalin monotherapy on fibromyalgia pain (81). The trial included an open-label pregabalin treatment period in which all patients received six weeks of pregabalin treatment (300, 450, or 600 mg/day). In the double-blind phase, all patients who responded to pregabalin treatment were randomized to continue treatment (300, 450, or 600 mg/day) or receive placebo for an additional 26 weeks or until they experienced a loss of therapeutic response. Of the 1,051 patients (93% female) enrolled in the trial, 663 completed the open-label phase and were assessed for response. Of these patients, 566 were pregabalin responders who were randomized to double-blind treatment (287 randomized to placebo, 279 to pregabalin). On the basis of Kaplan–Meier estimates of time to event, significantly more patients on placebo [174 (61%)] lost therapeutic response compared with 90 (32%) pregabalin patients. All secondary efficacy endpoints, including the Patient Global Impression of Change, total Fibromyalgia Impact Questionnaire score, Overall Sleep Problems Index of the MOS Sleep Scale, the Multidimensional Assessment of Fatigue, and the SF-36 Physical and Mental component scores, showed significantly greater time to loss of therapeutic response for pregabalin compared with placebo. The most frequently reported adverse events during the open-label treatment were dizziness (36%), somnolence (22%), headache (14%), and weight gain (11%).

Summary. The results of randomized, controlled trials of pregabalin in fibromyalgia demonstrate that pregabalin monotherapy reduces pain and improves other key symptom domains of fibromyalgia, such as sleep, and is associated with improvement in function, health-related quality of life, and global assessments. Pregabalin dosed at 150 mg BID, 225 mg BID, and 300 mg BID has a durable effect for maintaining patient's improvement in pain associated with fibromyalgia as well as in measures of global assessment, sleep, fatigue, and functional status in those who respond to pregabalin.

Gabapentin
Another $\alpha2$-δ ligand, gabapentin, is indicated by the FDA for adjunct therapy in adults with partial seizures and for postherpetic neuralgia (83). A multicenter, randomized, placebo-controlled, 12-week monotherapy trial tested the safety and efficacy of gabapentin 1200 to 2400 mg/day, administered three times daily, in

150 (90% female) patients with fibromyalgia (82). The primary outcome, the Brief Pain Inventory average pain severity score, significantly improved with gabapentin (median dose 1800 mg/day) compared with placebo (Table 3). Significantly more gabapentin-treated patients [38 (51%)] compared with placebo-treated patients [23 (31%)] experienced a response to treatment, defined as a 30% or more reduction in pain from baseline to endpoint. Most adverse events were mild to moderate in severity. The side effects reported by at least 5% of the gabapentin-treated patients that were more common in the gabapentin group were headache, dizziness, sedation, somnolence, edema, lightheadedness, insomnia, diarrhea, asthenia, depression, flatulence, nervousness, weight gain, amblyopia, anxiety, and dry mouth.

Summary. The results of this randomized, controlled study demonstrated that gabapentin monotherapy 1200 to 2400 mg/day (TID), taken for up to 12 weeks, reduces pain and improves other important symptom domains of fibromyalgia including sleep. It is associated with improvement in functionality and global assessments.

Sedative Hypnotic Medication
Nonbenzodiazepines and Benzodiazepines
Many patients with fibromyalgia experience disrupted or nonrestorative sleep and benefit from treatment to improve sleep. The nonbenzodiazepine sedatives, zolpidem and zopiclone, improved sleep and daytime energy in patients with fibromyalgia in short-term studies, but did not improve pain (84–86). Therefore these medications have limited usefulness as monotherapy, but may possibly be combined with other treatments for fibromyalgia. More data on the long-term use of nonbenzodiazepines in fibromyalgia are needed. Another study found no significant benefit of the benzodiazepine, bromazepan, over placebo in the treatment of fibromyalgia (87).

Sodium Oxybate
Sodium oxybate is the sodium salt of gammahydroxybutyrate (GHB), a metabolite of GABA with marked sedative properties. An eight-week study of sodium oxybate monotherapy evaluated 4.5 g/day or 6 g/day taken in two equally divided doses (bedtime and 2.5–4 hours later) in 188 patients with fibromyalgia (88). The primary outcome, a composite of changes from baseline in three coprimary measures—pain visual analog scale from electronic diaries, the Fibromyalgia Impact Questionnaire, and the patient global assessment—improved significantly with both dosages of sodium oxybate compared with placebo. Both dosages were also significantly superior to placebo in improvement in sleep quality, but the tender point count improved only in the higher sodium oxybate dose compared to placebo. The most common side effects were nausea and dizziness. GHB is associated with a high likelihood of abuse, cases of date rape, and, along with pentobarbital and methaqualone, is more likely to be lethal at supratherapeutic doses than any of the other hypnotics (89,90). Because of the risk of abuse, sodium oxybate, which was granted an orphan drug status by the FDA for the treatment of cataplexy and excessive daytime sleepiness in patients with narcolepsy, is only available through a Risk Management Program that was designed to educate physicians and patients about the safe use of the drug and minimize potential diversion or abuse by limiting distribution through a central pharmacy (91). This risk management program appears to be effective

in preventing diversion and limiting abuse in patients with narcolepsy, although the evaluation of the program is ongoing. Safer alternatives for the management of insomnia in patients with fibromyalgia include low-dose tricyclic agents, and, more recently, the α2-δ ligands, pregabalin, or gabapentin, which have sedative properties and relieve pain.

Opiates

Intravenous administration of morphine in nine patients with fibromyalgia did not reduce pain intensity in a small, double-blind, placebo-controlled study (92). A four-year, nonrandomized study found that fibromyalgia patients taking opiates did not report significant reduction in pain at the four-year follow-up, and experienced increased depression in the last two years of the study (93). Despite the lack of data supporting the use of opiates in fibromyalgia, a survey of U.S. academic medical centers found that about 14% of fibromyalgia patients are treated with opiates (94). A recent Internet survey of over 2500 self-identified patients with fibromyalgia reported that opioids were among the most commonly used treatments for fibromyalgia (95). The use of opiates in fibromyalgia continues to be controversial, not only because of the lack of supportive efficacy data but also because of the abuse potential of opiates and the emerging evidence of opioid-induced hyperalgesia (96). Recent preclinical studies suggest that chronic use of opioids induces neuroadaptive changes mediated, in part, through the NK-1 receptor that result in enhancement of nociceptive input (97). The potential development of opioid-induced hyperalgesia might limit the usefulness of opioids in controlling chronic pain associated with fibromyalgia.

Tramadol

Tramadol is a novel analgesic with weak agonist activity at the μ-opiate receptor combined with dual serotonin and norepinephrine reuptake inhibition. A double-blind crossover study compared single-dose intravenous tramadol 100 mg with placebo in 12 patients with fibromyalgia. Patients receiving tramadol experienced a 20.6% reduction in pain compared with a 19.8% increase in pain in the placebo group (98). Another study of tramadol began with a three-week, open-label phase of tramadol 50 to 400 mg/day followed by a six-week double-blind phase in which only patients who tolerated tramadol and perceived benefit were enrolled (99). The primary measure of efficacy was the time to exit from the double-blind phase because of inadequate pain relief. A total of 100 patients with fibromyalgia were enrolled in the open-label phase; 69% tolerated and perceived benefit from tramadol and were randomized to tramadol or placebo. Significantly fewer patients on tramadol discontinued during the double-blind phase because of inadequate pain relief. Finally, a multicenter, double-blind, randomized, placebo-controlled, 91-day study examined the efficacy of the combination of tramadol (37.5 mg) and acetaminophen (325 mg) in 315 patients with fibromyalgia (100,101). Patients taking tramadol and acetaminophen (4 $\pm$ 1.8 tabs/day) were significantly more likely than placebo-treated subjects to continue treatment and experience an improvement in pain and physical function. Improvements in the SF-36 physical functioning, role-physical, bodily pain, and physical component summary scores were significantly greater in the tramadol/acetominophen than the placebo group. The most common side effects in the tramadol/acetaminophen group were nausea, dizziness, somnolence, and constipation. Although tramadol is currently marketed as an analgesic without scheduling under the Federal Controlled Substances Act, it should be used with caution because of case reports of classical opioid withdrawal with discontinuation and dose reduction and reports of abuse and dependence.

Anti-inflammatory Medications

The corticosteroid, prednisone, was found to be ineffective in fibromyalgia, and corticosteroids are not recommended in the treatment of fibromyalgia (102). Patients with fibromyalgia frequently use nonsteroidal anti-inflammatory drugs (NSAIDs) or acetaminophen, although there is no evidence from clinical trials that they are effective when used alone in the treatment of fibromyalgia, and patients typically report that they offer minimal relief of pain. In one randomized, controlled trial, ibuprofen 600 mg four times daily was not more effective than placebo in reducing pain associated with fibromyalgia (103). The lack of a known significant inflammatory component in the pathophysiology of fibromyalgia may explain the poor response of fibromyalgia to NSAID monotherapy. However, studies have documented some benefit of ibuprofen and naproxen when combined with tricyclics (e.g., amitriptyline, cyclobenzaprine) or benzodiazepines (104–106). Fibromyalgia patients with a peripheral pain generator that could be aggravating fibromyalgia, such as comorbid osteoarthritis or other painful inflammatory conditions, would likely benefit from the addition of anti-inflammatory medications in the management of their pain.

CONCLUSIONS AND RECOMMENDATIONS FOR THE PHARMACOLOGICAL TREATMENT OF FIBROMYALGIA

The rapid growth of trials in fibromyalgia in recent years has resulted in new, evidence-based approaches to pharmacological treatment (107) (Table 4). Recent evidence suggests that comorbidity and the presence and severity of symptom domains should be an important consideration when selecting initial medication

TABLE 4 Summary of Key Findings from Pharmacological Studies in Fibromyalgia

1. SNRIs improve pain, other symptom domains, function, quality of life, and global well-being in patients with fibromyalgia
2. Selective SNRIs offer an alternative to cyclic medications (e.g., TCAs) that are associated with safety and tolerability concerns
3. The effects of SNRIs on reduction in pain associated with fibromyalgia are independent of their influence on mood
4. SSRIs are less consistently effective in reducing pain
5. Selective norepinephrine reuptake inhibitors show promise in the treatment of pain and fatigue associated with fibromyalgia
6. α2-δ Ligands improve pain, sleep, other symptom domains, function, and global well-being in patients with fibromyalgia
7. Drugs associated with high risk of abuse and dependence should be avoided. Opiates may contribute to hyperalgesia if used chronically
8. Although studies are limited, combinations of medications (e.g., combination of an SNRI and α2-δ ligand) may be an option for patients who do not fully respond to a single agent or who have problems with tolerability at higher doses

Abbreviations: SNRIs, serotonin and norepinephrine reuptake inhibitors; SSRIs, selective serotonin reuptake inhibitors.
Source: Adapted from Ref. (107).

TABLE 5 Recommendations for the Pharmacological Treatment of Fibromyalgia

Identify important symptom domains and their severity (e.g., pain, sleep disturbance, fatigue) and level of function

Evaluate for comorbid medical and psychiatric disorders (e.g., sleep apnea, osteoarthritis, depressive, or anxiety disorders); may require referral to specialist

Recommend treatment based on the results of the individual evaluation

    For patients with moderate to severe pain, trial with medication as a first-line approach:

        With or without lifetime depression or anxiety: trial of selective SNRI (not recommended as monotherapy for patients with comorbid bipolar disorder)

        Prominent sleep disturbance or anxiety: trial of α2-δ ligand

        Partial response to monotherapy with either SNRI or α2-δ ligand: trial of combination of these agents

        Consider other medications if no response to the above approach [e.g., SSRI; TCA; combination of SSRI with low dose TCA (watch for drug interaction between SSRI and TCA); combination of SSRI and α2-δ ligand]

        Avoid drugs with high likelihood of abuse or dependence

    Provide any additional treatment for comorbid conditions (e.g., NSAIDs for osteoarthritis, CPAP for sleep apnea)

Abbreviations: SNRI, serotonin and norepinephrine reuptake inhibitor; SSRI, selective serotonin reuptake inhibitors; NSAIDs, nonsteroidal anti-inflammatory drugs; CPAP, continuous positive airway pressure.
Source: Adapted from Ref. (107).

treatments for fibromyalgia. Until recently, a trial of tricyclic antidepressants or cyclobenzaprine was the first line approach to the medication treatment of fibromyalgia (28). However, these medications are often poorly tolerated and at low doses, are not effective for the treatment of mood or anxiety disorders, two common comorbid conditions. An alternative approach would be to recommend one of the new selective SNRIs as a first line treatment for pain in patients with or without depression or anxiety. One caveat related to the use of SNRIs or other medications with antidepressant effects in fibromyalgia is that they should not be used as monotherapy in patients with bipolar disorder, another frequently reported comorbid condition (108), because of the risk of increased mood instability. An alternative first line medication approach is an α2-δ ligand, which may be particularly helpful in patients with prominent sleep disturbances or anxiety. For those patients who do not respond completely to monotherapy with either an SNRI or an α2-δ ligand, a combination of these medications should be considered, although studies of this and other combination pharmacotherapy are still very limited (109). More recent work will likely expand the pharmacological treatment options for patients with fibromyalgia. For example, there are preliminary results for an NRI, which improves pain as well as fatigue, a common symptom in patients with fibromyalgia.

    Table 5 summarizes an approach to the pharmacological treatment of fibromyalgia, based on currently available medical evidence.

REFERENCES

1. Wolfe F, Smythe HA, Yunus MB, et al. The American College of Rheumatology 1990 criteria for the classification of fibromyalgia. Report of the Multicenter Criteria Committee. Arthritis Rheum 1990; 33:160–172.
2. Cleeland CS, Ryan KM. Pain assessment: global use of the brief pain inventory. Ann Acad Med Singapore 1994; 23:129–138.

3. Smets EM, Garssen B, Bonke B, et al. The Multidimensional Fatigue Inventory (MFI) psychometric qualities of an instrument to assess fatigue. J Psychosom Res 1995; 39: 315–325.

4. Belza B, Henke C, Epstein W, et al. Correlates of fatigue in older adults with rheumatoid arthritis. Nurs Res 1993; 42:93–99.

5. Hays RD, Stewart AL. Sleep measures. In: Stewart AL, Ware JEJ, eds. Measuring Functioning and Well-Being. Durham (NC): Duke University Press, 1992:232–259.

6. Hamilton M. A rating scale for depression. J Neurol Neurosurg Psychiatry 1960; 23: 56–62.

7. Zigmond A, Snaith RP. The hospital anxiety and depression scale. Acta Psychiatr Scand 1983; 67:361–370.

8. Seidenberg M, Haltiner A, Taylor MA, et al. Development and validation of a Multiple Ability Self-Report Questionnaire. J Clin Exp Neuropsychol 1994; 16: 93–104.

9. Fischer AA. Pressure threshold meter: its use for quantification of tender spots. Arch Phys Med Rehabil 1986; 67:836–838.

10. Burckhardt CS, Clark SR, Bennett RM. The Fibromyalgia Impact Questionnaire: development and validation. J Rheumatol 1991; 18:728–734.

11. Ware JE, Sherbourne CD. The SF-36 health status survey: I. Conceptual framework and item selection. Med Care 1992; 30:473–483.

12. Sheehan DV, Harnett-Sheehan K, Raj BA. The measurement of disability. Int Clin Psychopharmacol 1996; 11(suppl 3):89–95.

13. Hunt SM, McKenna SP. The QLDS: a scale for the measurement of quality of life in depression. Health Policy 1992; 22:307–319.

14. Kind P. The EuroQoL instrument: an index of health-related quality of life. In: Spilker B, ed. Quality of Life and Pharmacoeconomics in Clinical Trials. Philadelphia, PA: Lippincott-Raven Publishers, 1996:191–201.

15. Guy W. ECDEU Assessment Manual for Psychopharmacology, revised. US. Department of Health, Education, and Welfare publication (ADM). Rockville, MD: National Institute of Mental Health, 1976:76–338.

16. Pillemer SR, Bradley LA, Crofford LJ, et al. The neuroscience and endocrinology of fibromyalgia. Arthritis Rheum 1997; 40:1928–1939.

17. Lautenbacher S, Rollman GB. Possible deficiencies of pain modulation in fibromyalgia. Clin J Pain 1997; 13:189–196.

18. Bennett RM. Emerging concepts in the neurobiology of chronic pain: evidence of abnormal sensory processing in fibromyalgia. Mayo Clin Proc 1999; 74:385–398.

19. Staud, R. Evidence of involvement of central neural mechanisms in generating fibromyalgia pain. Curr Rheumatol Rep 2002; 4:299–305.

20. Basbaum AI, Fields HL. Endogenous pain control systems: brainstem spinal pathways and endorphin circuitry. Annu Rev Neurosci 1984; 7:309–338.

21. Clark FM, Proudfit HK. The projections of noradrenergic neurons in the A5 catecholamine cell group to the spinal cord in the rat: anatomical evidence that A5 neurons modulate nociception. Brain Res 1993; 616:200–210.

22. Millan MJ. Descending control of pain. Prog Neurobiol 2002; 66:355–474.

23. Russell IJ, Vaeroy H, Javors M, et al. Cerebrospinal fluid biogenic amine metabolites in fibromyalgia/fibrositis syndrome and rheumatoid arthritis. Arthritis Rheum 1992; 35:550–556.

24. Russell IJ, Michalek JE, Vipraio GA, et al. Platelet 3H-imipramine uptake receptor density and serum serotonin levels in patients with fibromyalgia/fibrositis syndrome. J Rheumatol 1992; 19:104–109.

25. Yunus MB, Dailey JW, Aldag JC, et al. Plasma tryptophan and other amino acids in primary fibromyalgia: a controlled study. J Rheumatol 1992; 19:90–94.

26. Coderre TJ, Katz J. Peripheral and central hyperexcitability: differential signs and symptoms in persistent pain. Behav Brain Sci 1997; 20:404–219.

27. Legangneux E, Mora JJ, Spreux-Varoquaux O, et al. Cerebrospinal fluid biogenic amine metabolites, plasma-rich platelet serotonin and [^{3}H]imipramine reuptake in the primary fibromyalgia syndrome. Rheumatology (Oxford) 2001; 40:290–296.

28. Fishbain DA, Cutler R, Rosomoff HL, et al. Evidence-based data from animal and human experimental studies on pain relief with antidepressants: a structured review. Pain Med 2000; 1:310–316.
29. Arnold LM. Duloxetine and other antidepressants in the treatment of patients with fibromyalgia. Pain Med 2007; 8(S2):63–74.
30. Arnold LM, Keck PE Jr., Welge JA. Antidepressant treatment of fibromyalgia. A meta-analysis and review. Psychosomatics 2000; 41:104–113.
31. Carette S, McCain GA, Bell DA, et al. Evaluation of amitriptyline in primary fibrositis: a double-blind, placebo-controlled study. Arthritis Rheum 1986; 29:655–659.
32. Carette S, Bell MJ, Reynolds WJ, et al. Comparison of amitriptyline, cyclobenzaprine, and placebo in the treatment of fibromyalgia: a randomized, double-blind clinical trial. Arthritis Rheum 1994; 37:32–40.
33. Carette S, Oakson G, Guimont C, et al. Sleep electroencephalography and the clinical response to amitriptyline in patients with fibromyalgia. Arthritis Rheum 1995; 38: 1211–1217.
34. Goldenberg DL, Mayskiy M, Mossey C, et al. A randomized double-blind crossover trial of fluoxetine and amitriptyline in the treatment of fibromyalgia. Arthritis Rheum 1996; 39:1852–1859.
35. Caruso I, Puttini PCS, Boccassini L, et al. Double-blind study of dothiepin versus placebo in the treatment of primary fibromyalgia syndrome. J Int Med Res 1987; 15:154–159.
36. Bennett RM, Gatter RA, Campbell SM, et al. A comparison of cyclobenzaprine and placebo in the management of fibrositis. Arthritis Rheum 1988; 31:1535–1542.
37. Quimby LG, Gratwick GM, Whitney CD, et al. A randomized trial of cyclobenzaprine for the treatment of fibromyalgia. J Rheumatol 1989; 16(suppl 19):140–143.
38. Reynolds WJ, Moldofsky H, Saskin P, et al. The effects of cyclobenzaprine on sleep physiology and symptoms in patients with fibromyalgia. J Rheumatol 1991; 18:452–454.
39. Kobayashi H, Hasegawa Y, One H. Cyclobenzaprine, a centrally acting muscle relaxant, acts on descending serotonergic systems. Eur J Pharmacol 1996; 311:29–35.
40. Bibolotti E, Borghi C, Pasculli E, et al. The management of fibrositis: a double-blind comparison of maprotiline (Ludiomil), chlorimipramine, and placebo. J Clin Trials 1986; 23:269–280.
41. Tofferi JK, Jackson JL, O'Malley PG. Treatment of fibromyalgia with cyclobenzaprine: a meta-analysis. Arthritis Rheum 2004; 51:9–13.
42. Goldenberg DL, Burckhardt C, Crofford L. Management of fibromyalgia syndrome. JAMA 2004; 292:2388–2395.
43. Beliles K, Stoudemire A. Psychopharmacologic treatment of depression in the medically ill. Psychosomatics 1998; 39:S2–S19.
44. Harvey AT, Rudolph RL, Preskorn SH. Evidence of the dual mechanisms of action of venlafaxine. Arch Gen Psychiatry 2000; 57:503–509.
45. Dwight MM, Arnold LM, O'Brien H, et al. An open clinical trial of venlafaxine in fibromyalgia. Psychosomatics 1998; 39:14–17.
46. Zijlstra TR, Barendregt PJ, van de Laar MAF. Venlafaxine in fibromyalgia: results of a randomized, placebo-controlled, double-blind trial. The 66th Annual Meeting of the American College of Rheumatology, New Orleans, LA, October 24–29, 2002.
47. Bymaster FP, Dreshfield-Ahmad LJ, Threlkeld PG, et al. Comparative affinity of duloxetine for serotonin and norepinephrine transporters in vitro and in vivo, human serotonin receptor subtypes, and other neuronal receptors. Neuropsychopharmacology 2001; 25:871–880.
48. Goldstein DJ, Mallinckrodt C, Lu Y, et al. Duloxetine in the treatment of major depressive disorder: a double-blind clinical trial. J Clin Psychiatry 2002; 63:225–231.
49. Detke MJ, Lu Y, Goldstein DJ, et al. Duloxetine 60 mg once daily for major depressive disorder: a randomized double-blind placebo-controlled trial. J Clin Psychiatry 2002; 63:308–315.
50. Detke MJ, Lu Y, Goldstein DJ, et al. Duloxetine 60 mg once daily dosing versus placebo in the acute treatment of major depression. J Psychiatr Res 2002; 36:383–390.
51. Goldstein DJ, Lu Y, Detke MJ, et al. Effects of duloxetine on painful physical symptoms associated with depression. Psychosomatics 2004; 45:17–28.

52. Raskin J, Pritchett YL, Wang F, et al. A double-blind, randomized multicenter trial comparing duloxetine with placebo in the management of diabetic peripheral neuropathic pain. Pain Med 2005; 6:346–356.
53. Goldstein DJ, Lu Y, Detke MJ, et al. Duloxetine vs. placebo in patients with painful diabetic neuropathy. Pain 2005; 116:109–118.
54. Eli Lilly and Company, Cymbalta (duloxetine), package insert. Indianapolis, IN, June 2008.
55. Arnold LM, Lu Y, Crofford LJ, et al. A double-blind, multicenter trial comparing duloxetine to placebo in the treatment of fibromyalgia patients with or without major depressive disorder. Arthritis Rheum 2004; 50:2974–2984.
56. Arnold LM, Rosen A, Pritchett YL, et al. A randomized, double-blind, placebo-controlled trial of duloxetine in the treatment of women with fibromyalgia with or without major depressive disorder. Pain 2005; 119:5–15.
57. Russell IJ, Mease PJ, Smith TR, et al. Efficacy and safety of duloxetine for treatment of fibromyalgia in patients with or without major depressive disorder: results from a 6-month, randomized, double-blind, placebo-controlled, fixed-dose trial. Pain 2008; 136: 432–444.
58. Gendreau RM, Thorn MD, Gendreau JF, et al. Efficacy of milnacipran in patients with fibromyalgia. J Rheumatol 2005; 32:1975–1985.
59. Mease PJ, Clauw DJ, Gendreau M, et al. The efficacy and safety of milnacipran for the treatment of fibromyalgia. Results of a randomized, double-blind, placebo-controlled trial. J Rheumatol 2009; 36(2):398–409.
60. Gahimer J, Wernicke J, Yalcin I, et al. A retrospective pooled analysis of duloxetine safety in 23, 983 subjects. Curr Med Res Opin 2007; 23:175–184.
61. Greist J, McNamara RK, Mallinckrodt CH, et al. Incidence and duration of antide-pressant-induced nausea: duloxetine compared with paroxetine and fluoxetine. Clin Ther 2004; 26:1446–1455.
62. Wernicke JF, Lledo A, Raskin J, et al. An evaluation of the cardiovascular safety profile of duloxetine: findings from 42 placebo-controlled studies. Drug Saf 2007; 30: 437–455.
63. Kranzler JD, Gendreau JF, Rao SG. The psychopharmacology of fibromyalgia: a drug development perspective. Psychopharmacol Bull 2002; 36:165–213.
64. Nørregaard J, Volkmann H, Danneskiold-Samsoe B. A randomized controlled trial of citalopram in the treatment of fibromyalgia. Pain 1995; 61:445–449.
65. Anderberg UM, Marteinsdottir I, von Knorring L. Citalopram in patients with fibromyalgia—a randomized, double-blind, placebo-controlled study. Eur J Pain 2000; 4:27–35.
66. Wolfe F, Cathey MA, Hawley DJ. A double-blind placebo controlled trial of fluox-etine in fibromyalgia. Scand J Rheumatol 1994; 23:255–259.
67. Arnold LM, Hess EV, Hudson JI, et al. A randomized, placebo-controlled, double-blind, flexible-dose study of fluoxetine in the treatment of women with fibro-myalgia. Am J Med 2002; 112:191–197.
68. Patkar AA, Masand PS, Krulewicz S, et al. A randomized, controlled trial of con-trolled release paroxetine in fibromyalgia. Am J Med 2007; 120:448–454.
69. Bymaster FP, Zhang W, Carter PA, et al. Fluoxetine, but not other selective serotonin uptake inhibitors, increases norepinephrine and dopamine extracellular levels in prefrontal cortex. Psychopharmacology 2002; 160:353–361.
70. Nemeroff CB, Owens MJ. Neuropharmacology of paroxetine. Psychopharmacol Bull 2003; 37(suppl 1):8–18.
71. Arnold LM, Chatamra K, Hirsch I, et al. Safety and efficacy of esreboxetine administered once daily in patients with fibromyalgia: an 8-week, randomized, double-blind, placebo-controlled, multicenter study. 72nd Annual Meeting of the American College of Rheumatology, San Francisco, CA, October 24–29, 2008.
72. Holman AJ, Myers RR. A randomized, double-blind, placebo-controlled trial of pramipexole, a dopamine agonist, in patients with fibromyalgia receiving con-comitant medications. Arthritis Rheum 2005; 52:2495–2505.

73. Woolf CJ. Pain: moving from symptom control toward mechanism-specific pharmacologic management. Ann Intern Med 2004; 140:441–451.
74. Dooley DJ, Taylor CP, Donevan S, et al. Ca^{2+} channel $\alpha_2\delta$ ligands: novel modulators of neurotransmission. Trends Pharmacol Sci 2007; 28:75–82.
75. Field MJ, Cox PJ, Stott E, et al. Identification of the alpha2-delta-1 subunit of voltage-dependent calcium channels as a molecular target for pain mediating the analgesic actions of pregabalin. Proc Natl Acad Sci U S A 2006; 103:17537–17542.
76. Taylor CP, Angelotti T, Fauman E. Pharmacology and mechanism of action of pregabalin: the calcium channel α_2-δ (alpha$_2$-delta) subunit as a target for antiepileptic drug discovery. Epilepsy Res 2007; 73:137–150.
77. Pfizer Inc, Lyrica (pregabalin), package insert. New York, NY; June 2007.
78. Crofford LJ, Rowbotham MC, Mease PJ, et al. Pregabalin for the treatment of fibromyalgia syndrome. Results of a randomized, double-blind, placebo-controlled trial. Arthritis Rheum 2005; 52:1264–1273.
79. Mease PJ, Russell IJ, Arnold LM, et al. A randomized, double-blind, placebo-controlled, phase III trial of pregabalin in the treatment of patients with fibromyalgia. J Rheumatol 2008; 35:502–514.
80. Arnold LM, Russell IJ, Diri EW, et al. A 14-week, randomized, double-blinded, placebo-controlled monotherapy trial of pregabalin in patients with fibromyalgia. J Pain 2008; 9:792–805.
81. Crofford LJ, Mease PJ, Simpson SL, et al. Fibromyalgia relapse evaluation and efficacy for durability of meaningful relief (FREEDOM): a 6-month, double-blind, placebo-controlled trial with pregabalin. Pain 2008; 136:419–431.
82. Arnold LM, Goldenberg DL, Stanford SB, et al. Gabapentin in the treatment of fibromyalgia. A randomized, double-blind, placebo-controlled, multicenter trial. Arthritis Rheum 2007; 56:1336–1344.
83. Pfizer Inc, Neurontin (gabapentin), package insert. New York, NY; January 2007.
84. Drewes AM, Andreasen A, Jennum P, et al. Zopiclone in the treatment of sleep abnormalities in fibromyalgia. Scand J Rheumatol 1991; 20:288–293.
85. Grönblad M, Nykänen J, Konttinen Y, et al. Effect of zopiclone of sleep quality, morning stiffness, widespread tenderness and pain and general discomfort in primary fibromyalgia patients. A double-blind randomized trial. Clin Rheumatol 1993; 12:186–191.
86. Moldofsky H, Lue FA, Mously C, et al. The effect of zolpidem in patients with fibromyalgia: a dose ranging, double-blind, placebo controlled, modified crossover study. J Rheumatol 1996; 23:529–533.
87. Quijada-Carrera J, Valenzuela-Castano A, Povedano-Gomez J, et al. Comparison of tenoxicam and bromazepan in the treatment of fibromyalgia: a randomized, double-blind, placebo-controlled trial. Pain 1996; 65:221–225.
88. Russell IJ, Bennett RM, Michalek JE. Oxybate for FMS Study Group: Sodium oxybate relieves pain and improves sleep in fibromyalgia syndrome [FMS]: a randomized, double-blind, placebo-controlled, multi-center clinical trial. 69th Annual Meeting of the American College of Rheumatology, San Diego, CA, November 12–17, 2005.
89. Nicholson KL, Balster RL. GHB: a new and novel drug of abuse. Drug Alcohol Depend 2001; 63:1–22.
90. Griffiths RR, Johnson MW. Relative abuse liability of hypnotic drugs: a conceptual framework and algorithm for differentiating among compounds. J Clin Psychiatry 2005; 66(suppl 9):31–41.
91. Fuller DE, Hornfeldt CS, Kelloway JS, et al. The Xyrem® risk management program. Drug Saf 2004; 27:293–306.
92. Sorensen J, Bengtsson A, Backman E, et al. Pain analysis in patients with fibromyalgia. Effects of intravenous morphine, lidocaine, and ketamine. Scand J Rheumatol 1995; 24:360–365.
93. Kemple KL, Smith G, Wong-Ngan J. Opioid therapy in fibromyalgia- a four year prospective evaluation of therapy selection, efficacy, and predictors of outcome. Arthritis Rheum 2003; 48:S88.

94. Wolfe F, Anderson J, Harkness D, et al. A prospective, longitudinal, multicenter study of service utilization and costs in fibromyalgia. Arthritis Rheum 1997; 40: 1560–1570.
95. Bennett RM, Jones J, Turk DC, et al. An internet survey of 2,596 people with fibromyalgia. BMC Musculoskelet Disord 2007; 8:27.
96. Chu LF, Clark DJ, Angst MS. Opioid tolerance and hyperalgesia in chronic pain patients after one month of oral morphine therapy: a preliminary prospective study. J Pain 2006; 7:43–48.
97. King T, Gardell LR, Wang R, et al. Role of NK-1 neurotransmission in opioid-induced hyperalgesia. Pain 2005; 116:276–288.
98. Biasi G, Manca S, Manganelli S, et al. Tramadol in the fibromyalgia syndrome: a controlled clinical trial versus placebo. Int J Clin Pharmacol Res 1998; 18:13–19.
99. Russell IJ, Kamin M, Bennett RM, et al. Efficacy of tramadol in treatment of pain in fibromyalgia. J Clin Rheumatol 2000; 6:250–257.
100. Bennett RM, Kamin M, Karim R, et al. Tramadol and acetaminophen combination tablets in the treatment of fibromyalgia pain: a double-blind, randomized, placebo-controlled study. Am J Med 2003; 114:537–545.
101. Bennett RM, Schein J, Kosinski MR, et al. Impact of fibromyalgia pain on health-related quality of life before and after treatment with tramadol/acetaminophen. Arthritis Rheum 2005; 53:519–527.
102. Clark S, Tindall E, Bennett RM. A double blind crossover trial of prednisone versus placebo in the treatment of fibrositis. J Rheumatol 1985; 12:980–983.
103. Yunus MB, Masi AT, Aldag JC. Short term effects of ibuprofen in primary fibromyalgia syndrome: a double blind, placebo-controlled trial. J Rheumatol 1989; 16: 527–532.
104. Goldenberg DL, Felson DT, Dinerman H. A randomized, controlled trial of amitriptyline and naproxen in the treatment of patients with fibromyalgia. Arthritis Rheum 1986; 29:1371–1377.
105. Fossaluzza V, De Vita S. Combined therapy with cyclobenzaprine and ibuprofen in primary fibromyalgia syndrome. Int J Clin Pharmacol Res 1992; 12:99–102.
106. Russell IJ, Fletcher EM, Michalek JE, et al. Treatment of primary fibrositis/fibromyalgia syndrome with ibuprofen and alprazolam. A double-blind, placebo-controlled study. Arthritis Rheum 1991; 34:552–560.
107. Arnold LM. Biology and therapy of fibromyalgia. New therapies in fibromyalgia. Arthritis Res Ther 2006; 8:212.
108. Arnold LM, Hudson JI, Keck PE Jr., et al. Comorbidity of fibromyalgia and psychiatric disorders. J Clin Psychiatry 2006; 67:1219–1225.
109. Arnold LM. Systemic therapies for chronic pain. In: Wallace DJ, Clauw DJ, eds. Fibromyalgia and Other Central Pain Syndromes. Philadelphia, PA: Lippincott Williams & Wilkins, 2005:365–388.

5 Psychosocial Issues in Fibromyalgia

Dennis C. Turk and Hilary D. Wilson
Department of Anesthesiology, University of Washington, Seattle, Washington, U.S.A.

INTRODUCTION

The view that psychological factors and emotion states generate or exacerbate pain has a long and colorful history as illustrated by Tuke's (1) account of the case of a terrified butcher, who on trying to hook up a piece of meat, slipped, was suspended by the arm on the hook, and when taken to a chemist, said he suffered acute agony. The hook had only transversed his coat and the arm was uninjured, and yet through fear he cried out with "excessive pain" when the sleeve was cut off in order to let his arm be examined. Was the butcher's pain real? Was it all psychogenic? Did some preexisting psychopathology predispose the butcher to interpret the situation in the way he did? Is he just a malingering who wished to use his accident as a way to obtain time off from his onerous job?

There has been an ongoing debate in the fibromyalgia (FM) syndrome literature as to whether psychological factors are causal or a reaction to the presence of a large number of symptoms with unknown cause and no cure. For example, some have suggested that FM is one of a set of depression spectrum disorders (2), whereas others note that the lifetime prevalence of psychiatric disorders is high in FM (3–5), yet not all patients will have a significant psychiatric history. For example, a study of a community sample of patients with FM showed that depressive and anxiety symptoms were often severe with about one-third of these individuals reporting major current problem with depression or anxiety (6). Moreover, given the heterogeneity of patients both in the number and nature of their symptoms, perceived cause, and differential patterns of adaptation, it is reasonable to assume that FM is not a homogeneous diagnostic classification. We will illustrate this later in the chapter. Depending on unique characteristics, different treatments may have to be matched to patient subgroups that differ in important ways despite the common diagnosis.

The debate as to whether FM is a syndrome caused by psychological factors—is psychogenic—or a set of symptoms with a physical basis but with the subsequent development of emotional distress in response, therefore somatopsychic, may be of theoretical interest and we will return to this later in this chapter. Regardless of the cause or effect relationship, when treating patients both physical and emotional symptoms need to be assessed and addressed.

It is important to make a distinction between psychological causation of symptoms and disease onset and psychosocial factors as mediators and moderators of persistent symptoms, adaptation, response to symptoms and treatments. Any chronic disease has an impact on all domains of people's lives and not just their bodies. This is true whether we are speaking of diabetes, end-stage renal disease, asthma, rheumatoid arthritis (RA), or FM. In each case symptoms persist despite treatment, affect daily functioning, and consequently require significant degrees of self-management beyond medical care. Moreover, people with FM have unique personal histories and genetic composition. The average

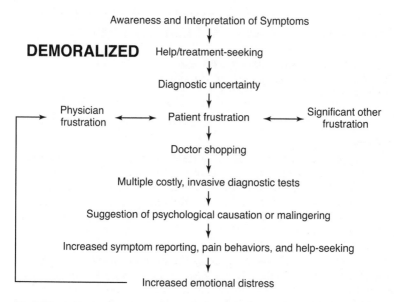

Awareness and Interpretation of Symptoms
↓
DEMORALIZED   Help/treatment-seeking
↓
Diagnostic uncertainty
↓
Physician   ←→   Patient frustration   ←→   Significant other
frustration   frustration
↓
Doctor shopping
↓
Multiple costly, invasive diagnostic tests
↓
Suggestion of psychological causation or malingering
↓
Increased symptom reporting, pain behaviors, and help-seeking
↓
Increased emotional distress

FIGURE 1   Natural history of persistent symptoms: A patients' perspective.

age of FM patients seen in our treatment center is 44, and the duration of symptoms exceeds seven years by the time of their initial evaluation. Thus, these patients have had 37 years of history that will affect their symptom presentation, response, and adaptation. By the time they are referred to our tertiary care facility they have been living with their symptoms for an average of seven years. In a large Internet-based survey, 25% of all responders had seen more than six healthcare providers in a search to obtain a diagnosis, and their previous experience with healthcare providers is yet another part of their history that will affect their symptom presentation (7).

The patients we treat also live in a social context that will influence their situation. Seeking the cause for each symptom and prescribing a treatment for the many that are common to FM, in the absence of a cure, will lead to inadequate outcomes. Patients will continue to be frustrated, feeling helpless and hopeless as they are exposed to the litany of tests and treatments. Indeed, examination of the published literature reveals that over 100 pharmacological and nonpharmacological treatments have been reported to provide some beneficial effects, on some symptoms, for some patients. It is helpful to understand the plight of the FM patients by considering what they experience in their quest to obtain relief, which is outlined in Figure 1 and described in the following text.

THE EXPERIENCE OF PERSISTENT SYMPTOMS

For a person with FM, there is a continuing quest for relief that remains elusive and leads to feelings of frustration, demoralization, and depression, compromising the quality of all aspects of their lives. People with FM confront not only the stress of their symptoms but also a cascade of ongoing problems (e.g., financial, familial). Moreover, the experience of "medical limbo" (i.e., the presence of a painful condition that eludes diagnosis and that carries the implication of either psychiatric causation or malingering on the one hand, or an undiagnosed potentially disabling condition on the other) is itself a source of significant stress and can initiate psychological distress.

Regardless of the causes for the original symptoms, over time, psychosocial and behavioral factors may serve to maintain and exacerbate symptoms, influence adjustment, and contribute to excessive disability. Following from this view, pain and related symptoms of FM that persist over time should not be viewed as solely physical or solely psychological; the experience of pain is maintained by an interdependent set of biomedical, psychosocial, and behavioral factors.

Consider the following scenario. A woman with widespread pain, fatigue, and a range of other symptoms becomes inactive, leading to preoccupation with her body and pain, and these cognitive-attentional changes increase her likelihood of amplifying and distorting pain symptoms. She may begin to perceive herself as being disabled. At the same time, due to fear, she limits her opportunities to identify activities that build flexibility, endurance, and strength without the risk of pain or injury. To the person with FM, hurt is often viewed as synonymous with harm. Fatigue drives them to withdraw from activity and they lack energy and may fear that undertaking activity may exacerbate their symptoms. Thus, if an activity produces an increase in pain and fatigue, the person with FM terminates the activity and avoids similar activities in the future. Indeed, people with FM often develop negative expectations about their own ability to exert any control over their pain, fatigue, and related symptoms. The negative expectations lead to feelings of frustration and demoralization when "uncontrollable" symptoms interfere with participation in physical and social activities.

People with FM frequently terminate efforts to develop new strategies to manage pain and, instead, turn to passive coping strategies such as inactivity, medication, or alcohol to reduce emotional distress and the host of symptoms they experience. They also absolve themselves of personal responsibility for managing their symptoms and, instead, rely on family and healthcare providers. The thinking or "cognitive activity" of people with FM may contribute to the exacerbation, attenuation, or maintenance of pain, pain behaviors, affective distress, and dysfunctional adjustment to chronic pain.

Significant others also may unwittingly contribute to the disability observed in people with FM. For example, if the complaint of a person with FM about her pain and fatigue results in her husband giving her more attention, then this positive attention may reinforce and thereby increase the likelihood of more complaint to obtain the desired attention. The physician who responds to the patient's complaints of increased pain and fatigue by suggesting that "if it hurts do not do it" may be promoting complaints as a means for the patient to avoid pain and fatigue produced by the use of deconditioned muscles during physical activity.

If psychological factors can influence pain in a maladaptive manner, then they can also have a positive effect. People who feel that they have a number of successful methods for coping with symptoms may suffer less than those who feel helpless and hopeless.

In the case of FM, healthcare providers need to consider not only the physical basis of symptoms (the nociceptive, sensory component) but also patients' mood, fears, expectancies, coping resources, coping efforts, and response of significant others, including themselves. Regardless of whether there is an identifiable physical basis for the reported symptoms, psychosocial and behavioral factors will interact to influence the nature, severity, and persistence of pain and disability. In particular, behavioral, emotional, and cognitive variables should be addressed. We can now consider the specific psychological principles and variables and show how they may influence symptom perception, reports of symptoms, and response to treatment.

BEHAVIORAL FACTORS

Pain and fatigue are potent and salient experience for humans. We all attempt to avoid, modify, or cope with these negative sensations. There are three major principles of behavioral learning that help us understand acquisition of adaptive as well as dysfunctional behaviors associated with symptoms.

Classical (Respondent) Conditioning

Classical conditioning is widely known as Pavlovian learning from the research of the Russian physiologist, Ivan Pavlov. In his classic experiment, Pavlov found that a dog could be taught, or "conditioned," to salivate at the sound of a bell by pairing the sound with food presented to a hungry dog. Salivation of dogs to food is a natural response; however, by preceding the feeding with the sound of a bell, Pavlov's dogs *learned* to associate the bell with an imminent feeding. Once this association was learned or conditioned the dogs were found to salivate at the mere sound of the bell *even in the absence of the food*. That is, the dogs were conditioned to anticipate food at the sound of a bell.

The influence of classical conditioning can be observed in humans as well as dogs. For example, cancer patients receiving chemotherapy often experience extreme gastrointestinal symptoms (nausea and vomiting) resulting from the pharmacological effects of chemotherapy. The nausea has been shown to be classically conditioned to neutral cues paired with the chemotherapy, such as doctors, nurses, the hospital, and even patients' clothes (8). Once acquired, learned responses tend to persist over long periods. It is common to observe cancer patients long in remission who report nausea when they see their doctor's face, even years after the completion of the treatment.

Lack of physical conditioning is frequently observed in people with FM and increases in exercise are among the most frequently recommended treatments. Despite the referral for physical therapy, many patients with FM resist or prematurely terminate participation in conditioning programs. Classical conditioning is likely one important contributor to nonadherence to exercise recommendations. Table 1 illustrates the way in which physical therapists may evoke a conditioned fear response in the FM patients they are treating.

TABLE 1　Classical Conditioning: Example with Pain-Exercise Association

Step 1: Natural Consequence of Pain—
　　　　Fear
　　　　PAIN ↑ FEAR
Step 2: Pairing Exercise
　　　　↑ FEAR
　　　　PAIN
Step 3: Conditioned Fear
　　　　Exercise ↑ FEAR

A patient, for example, who received treatment that intensified symptoms may become conditioned to experience a negative emotional response to the presence of the healthcare provider, to the treatment room, and to any contextual cues associated with the nociceptive stimulus. The negative emotional reaction may lead to tensing of muscles and this in turn may exacerbate symptoms and thereby strengthen the association between the presence of the physical therapist and pain.

Once symptoms persist, fear of motor activities becomes increasingly conditioned, resulting in avoidance of activity. The avoidance of pain and fatigue are powerful rationale for reduction of activity, whereas muscle soreness associated with exercise functions as a justification for further avoidance. Thus, although it may be useful to reduce movement in the acute stage, limitation of activities can be chronically maintained not only by symptoms but also by anticipatory fear that has been acquired through classical conditioning. This may be an important explanation for the high premature termination rates of FM patients with prescribed physical therapy regimens. We have often heard patients protest that although they know they should be more active, "I'll pay for it tomorrow." Here it is the anticipation of aversive consequences that impedes engagement in physical exercise programs.

In FM, many activities that are neutral or pleasurable may elicit or exacerbate symptoms and are thus experienced as aversive and are avoided. Over time, more and more activities (e.g., people, physical locations, physical exercise) may be expected to elicit or exacerbate symptoms and will be avoided. Anticipation of symptom flare-ups may become associated with an expanding number of situations and behaviors. Avoided activities may involve simple motor behaviors but may also involve work, leisure, and sexual activity. Anticipatory fear and anxiety also elicit physiological reactivity that may aggravate symptoms. Thus, psychological factors may directly affect nociceptive stimulation and need not be viewed as only reactions to symptoms.

Insofar as activity avoidance succeeds in preventing symptom aggravation, the conviction that patients should remain inactive will be difficult to modify. By contrast, repeatedly engaging in behavior that produces significantly less pain and fatigue than was predicted (corrective feedback) will be followed by reductions in anticipatory fear and anxiety associated with the activity. These adjustments will be increasingly followed by appropriate avoidance behavior, even to elimination of all inappropriate avoidance. Such transformations add support to the importance of a quota-based physical therapy program, with patients progressively increasing their activity levels despite fear of injury and discomfort associated with renewed use of deconditioned muscles.

Operant Conditioning: Environmental Contingencies of Reinforcement

A new era in thinking about pain began in 1976 with Fordyce's (9) extension of *operant conditioning* to chronic pain. The main focus of operant learning is modification in frequency of a given behavior. If the consequence of the given behavior is rewarding, the likelihood of its occurrence increases; if the consequence is aversive, the likelihood of its occurrence decreases (Table 2). Thus, only preexisting behaviors are conditioned.

Behaviors associated with symptoms, such as distorted ambulation, rubbing painful body parts, lying down during the day, are called "symptom

TABLE 2 Operant Schedules of Reinforcement

Schedule	Consequences	Probability of the behavior recurring
Positive reinforcement	Reward the behavior	More likely
Negative reinforcement	Prevent or withdraw aversive results	More likely
Punishment	Punish the behavior	Less likely
Neglect	Prevent or withdraw positive results	Less likely

behaviors." When a person is exposed to a stimulus that causes tissue damage, the immediate behavior is withdrawal in an attempt to escape from noxious sensations. Such symptom behaviors are adaptive and appropriate. According to Fordyce (9), these behaviors can be subjected to the principles of operant conditioning. For example, symptom behaviors such as avoidance of activity and help-seeking effectively prevent or withdraw aversive results (e.g., pain, fatigue). This negative reinforcement makes such behaviors more likely to occur in the future. The operant view proposes that acute symptom behaviors such as avoidance of activity to protect a wounded limb from producing additional noxious input may come under the control of external contingencies of reinforcement (responses increase or decrease as a function of their reinforcing consequences: Table 2), and thus develop into a chronic problem.

Symptom behaviors are conceptualized as overt expressions of symptoms, distress, and suffering. As we noted earlier, these behaviors may be positively reinforced directly, for example, by attention from a spouse or healthcare providers. The principles of learning suggest that behaviors that are positively reinforced will be reported more frequently. Symptom behaviors may also be maintained by the escape from noxious stimulation by the use of drugs or rest, or the avoidance of undesirable activities such as work. In addition "well behaviors" (e.g., activity, working) may not be positively reinforced, and the more rewarding symptom behaviors may therefore be maintained.

Consider an example to illustrate the role of operant conditioning. When a woman with symptoms of FM flares up, she may lie down to rest. Her husband may observe her behavior and infer that she is experiencing intensification of her symptoms. He may respond by offering to bring her some medication, to take children out to the park to give her quiet, or to assume some household chores such as washing the family's clothes. Such response may positively reward the woman, and her behaviors (i.e., lying down) may be repeated even in the absence of symptoms. In other words, the woman's symptom behaviors are being maintained by the learned consequences.

It should be noted that people with FM may not consciously communicate about their symptoms to obtain attention or to avoid undesirable activities. It is more likely to be the result of a gradual process of the shaping of behavior that neither she nor her husband recognizes. Thus a person's response to life stressors as well as how others respond to the person with FM can influence the experience of symptoms in many ways, but are not the initial cause of the symptoms.

Healthcare professionals may also reinforce symptoms by their responses. The physician who prescribes medication on the patient's complaint may be reinforcing the patient's reports of symptoms. That is, the patient learns that his

Operant Conditioning Stage: **Chronic Stage: even without symptoms**

Symptoms → Lying down → Sympathy (Positive Reinforcement)   → Sx likely to recur

Sx → Lying down → Avoiding work (Negative Reinforcement)   → Sx likely to recur

Sx → Exercise → Flare-up (Punishment)   → Exercise unlikely to recur

Sx → Exercise → Apathy from others (Neglect)   → Exercise unlikely to recur

FIGURE 2 Operant maintenance of symptom behavior in FM: Example.

or her behavior elicits a response from the physician, and if the response provides some relief, then the patient may learn to report pain in order to obtain the desired outcome. This is the case when pain medication is prescribed on a "take as needed" (*prn*) basis. In this case the patient must indicate that the pain has increased in order to take the medication. If the medication provides some reduction of symptoms then the attention to and self-rating of symptoms may be maintained by the anticipated outcome of relief. In several studies, the interaction of physicians and patients have been shown to unwittingly reinforce patients' symptom reporting by providing further attention and more intensive treatments based on patients' reports rather than any evidence of physical pathology (10,11).

Physical therapists who suggest that patients engage in some exercises until the "pain and fatigue become excessive" are functioning in the same way as the physician. The reinforcement of reduction in activity to reduce pain will come to maintain complaints and subsequently inactivity. The alternative for the physical therapist is to prescribe exercises on a work-to-goal rather than work-to-pain basis. Termination of the exercise is then paired with completion of a designated set of exercises, not pain. Here we can see how classical and operant conditionings become related. The pairing of the neutral and pain-evoking stimuli is classically conditioned, and the reinforcement schedule established by the healthcare professional leads to operant learning.

The combination of reinforced pain behaviors and neglected well behaviors is common in FM (Fig. 2). The operant learning paradigm does not uncover the etiology of symptoms but focuses primarily on the maintenance of symptom behaviors and deficiency in well behaviors. Operant technique focuses on the elimination of symptom behaviors by withdrawal of attention and increasing of well behaviors by positive reinforcement. The operant view has generated what has proven to be an effective treatment for select samples of FM patients (12,13).

Social Learning Mechanisms

Social learning has received some attention in acute pain and in the development and maintenance of chronic pain states. From this perspective, the acquisition of symptom behaviors may occur by means of "observational" learning and "modeling" processes. That is, people can acquire responses that were not previously in their behavioral repertoire by the observation of others performing these activities. Children acquire attitudes about health and healthcare, and the perception and interpretation of symptoms and physiological processes from their parents and social environment. They learn appropriate and inappropriate responses to injury and disease and thus may be more or less likely to ignore or overrespond to symptoms they experience based on behaviors modeled in childhood. The culturally acquired perception and interpretation of symptoms determines how people deal with illness.

Expectancies and actual behavioral responses to nociceptive stimulation are based, at least partially, on prior social learning history. This may contribute to the marked variability in response to objectively similar degrees of physical pathology noted by healthcare providers.

EMOTIONAL (AFFECTIVE) FACTORS

Symptoms such as pain and fatigue are ultimately subjective, private experiences, but they are invariably described in terms of sensory and affective properties. As defined by the International Association for the Study of Pain: "[Pain] is unquestionably a sensation in a part or parts of the body but it is also always unpleasant and therefore also an emotional experience" (14). The central and interactive roles of sensory information and affective state are supported by an overwhelming amount of evidence (15). The affective components of pain include many different emotions, but they are primarily negative emotions.

In addition to affect being one of the three interconnected components of pain, symptoms and emotions interact in a number of ways. Emotional distress may predispose people to experience symptoms, be a precipitant of symptoms, be a modulating factor amplifying or inhibiting the severity of symptoms, be a consequence of persistent symptoms, or be a perpetuating factor. Moreover, these potential roles are not mutually exclusive and any number of them may be involved in a particular circumstance interacting with cognitive appraisals.

Although we will provide an overview of research on the predominant emotions—anxiety, depression, and anger—associated with symptoms individually, it is important to acknowledge that these emotions are not as distinct when it comes to the experience of symptoms. They interact and augment each other over time.

Anxiety

Anxiety is commonplace in chronic pain. This is especially true when the symptoms are unexplained, as is often the case for FM. For example, in a large-scale, multicentered study of FM patients, between 44% and 51% patients acknowledged that they were anxious (16), and a recent epidemiological study comparing FM patients to healthcare users without FM claims indicated that FM patients were more than four times as likely to have an anxiety-related claim (17). People with FM may be anxious about the meaning of their symptoms and for their futures—will their symptoms increase, will their physical capacity diminish, will their symptoms result in progressive disability where they ultimately end in a wheelchair or are bedridden? In addition to these sources of fear, people with FM may be worried that, on the one hand, people will not believe that they are suffering and, on the other, they may be told that they are beyond help and will "just have to learn to live with it." Fear and anxiety will also relate to activities that people with FM anticipate will increase their pain and fatigue or exacerbate whatever physical factors might be contributing to their symptoms. These fears may contribute to avoidance, motivate inactivity, and ultimately greater disability.

Pain-related fear and concerns about harm avoidance appear to exacerbate symptoms (18). Anxiety is an affective state that is influenced by appraisal processes. To cite the stoic philosopher Epictetus, "There is nothing either bad or good but thinking makes it so." There is a reciprocal relationship between affective state and cognitive-interpretive processes whereby thinking affects mood and mood influences appraisals and ultimately the experience of pain.

Threat of intense pain captures attention and is difficult to disengage from. Continual vigilance and monitoring of noxious stimulation and the belief that it signifies disease progression may render even low-intensity nociception less bearable. As we noted in our discussion of respondent conditioning, the experience of pain may initiate a set of extremely negative thoughts and arouse fears—fears of inciting more pain, injury, and the future impact (19). Fear of pain and anticipation of pain are cognitive-perceptual processes that are not driven exclusively by the actual sensory experience of pain and can exert a significant impact on the level of function and pain tolerance (20). In a classic demonstration of the role of expectancy and fear, Bayer et al. (21) told 100 volunteers that they would receive an electrical shock that might possibly produce pain. The investigators did not explain that the shock stimulator device they were using was a sham, emitting nothing beyond a low humming sound. Over 50% of the patients reported pain, and the ratings of pain intensity increased as the participants observed the setting on the sham stimulator being increased by the experimenter.

Several investigators (18,22) have suggested that fear of pain, driven by the anticipation of pain rather than the sensory experience of pain, is a strong negative reinforcement for the persistence of avoidance behavior and functional disability. Avoidance behavior is reinforced in the short term through the reduction of suffering associated with nociception. Avoidance, however, can be a maladaptive response if it persists and leads to increased fear, limited activity, and other physical and psychological consequences that contribute to disability and persistence of pain (18,23).

Enduring psychological and functional limitation following a traumatic event is frequently indicative of "posttraumatic stress disorder" (PTSD). Traumatic events have been associated with a set of symptoms, including nightmares, recurrent and intrusive recollections about the trauma, avoidance of thoughts or activities associated with the traumatic event, and symptoms of increased arousal such as insomnia and hyperarousal. When this set of symptoms closely follows a known traumatic event over an extended period of time, they are labeled PTSD. Significant minorities of chronic pain sufferers attribute the onset of their symptoms to a specific trauma such as a motor vehicle accident. Results of research suggest an exceedingly high prevalence of PTSD in patients visiting chronic pain clinics (24), including FM patients (25–27) and community samples (28).

In a preliminary study, Sherman et al. (2000) (27) found that over 50% of a sample of 93 female, treatment-seeking FM patients reported symptoms of PTSD. Those who experienced these anxiety-related symptoms reported significantly greater levels of pain, life interference, emotional distress, and greater inactivity than did the patients who did not report PTSD-like symptoms. Over 85% of the sample with significant PTSD symptoms compared to 50% of the patients without significant PTSD symptoms demonstrated significant disability. Cohen et al. (26) also found that a similar proportion of both male and female FM patients had clinically significant levels of PTSD. More recently, Amital and colleagues (25) reported that 49% of male patients with PTSD subsequent to war-related trauma met the American College of Rheumatology (ACR) (16) criteria for FM. This can be compared with only 5% of patients with major depressive disorder who meet the ACR criteria. In a diverse community study of women, using a standard psychiatric interview (SCID) (29), Raphael et al. (28) found that the risk of PTSD was approximately fivefold higher among a sample of women with FM although the current level was virtually 0. Based on these results, clinicians should assess the presence of these symptoms, as the failure to attend to them in treatment may undermine successful outcomes.

Depression

Research suggests that from 40% to 50% of chronic pain patients are depressed (30). The incidence of depression among FM patients is even higher than observed in other chronic pain patients, ranging as high as 70% in clinic samples (5,31) and exceeding 30% in community samples (6). Although the epidemiological studies provide solid evidence for a strong association between chronic pain and depression, they do not address whether chronic pain causes depression or depression causes chronic pain. Prospective studies of patients with chronic musculoskeletal pain have suggested that chronic pain can cause depression (32), that depression can cause chronic pain (33), and that they exist in a mutually reinforcing relationship (34).

One fact often raised to support the idea that pain causes depression is that the current depressive episode often began following the onset of the pain problem. The majority of studies appear to support this contention (35). However, several studies have documented that many patients with chronic pain (especially those disabled patients seen in pain clinics) have often had prior episodes of depression that predated their pain problem by years (36). One important prospective study (37) demonstrated that levels of depression predicted the development of low back pain three years following the initial assessment. Patients with depression were 2.3 times more likely to report back pain compared to those who did not report depression. Depression was a much stronger predictor of incident back pain than any clinical or anatomic risk factor. This has led some investigators to propose that there may exist a common trait of susceptibility to dysphoric physical symptoms (including pain) and to negative psychological symptoms (including anxiety as well as depression). They conclude that "pain and psychological illness should be viewed as having reciprocal psychological and behavioral effects involving both processes of illness expression and adaptation" (38).

Another important issue is the economic costs of FM. These include direct healthcare costs and indirect costs associated with lost days of work, impairment of optimal work performance, disability cost, and lost tax revenue, too name only a few. The cost of FM has been shown to be twice as high for patients with FM ($5163) compared to a random sample of the overall beneficiary population ($2486), but more than 4.8 times higher for patients that are diagnosed with a combination of FM and depression ($11,899) (39). Thus, not only is FM costly, the combination of FM and depression greatly escalates the costs.

As noted previously, in majority of cases, depression appears to be reactive, although some have suggested that chronic pain is a form of "masked depression," whereby patients use pain to express their depressed mood because they feel it is more acceptable to complain of pain than to acknowledge that one is depressed. Once a person has a chronic pain diagnosis, it no longer matters which is the cause and which is the consequence—pain or depression. Both need to be treated.

Anger

Anger has been widely observed in patients with chronic pain (40,41). Chronic angry emotional reactions are often maladaptive because they lead to pervasive interpersonal disruption and conflict with significant others including healthcare providers, alter descending and central pain modulation systems, and lead to chronic sympathetic activation that may exacerbate symptoms (42).

Anger management style refers to the patterns people used to express or externalize anger, suppress or internalize anger, or control their anger. Kerns et al. (43) found that the internalization of angry feelings accounted for a significant proportion of variances in measures of pain intensity, perceived interference, and reported frequency of pain behaviors. Similarly, Okifuji et al. (44) noted that 70% of a clinic sample of chronic pain patients acknowledged having angry feelings directed toward someone or something when asked; even this high prevalence may be an underestimate due to denial by patients. Moreover, anger directed toward oneself was significantly associated with pain and depression. In the anonymous Internet survey (7), over 85% of people with FM acknowledged some degree of anger.

Elevated anger has been associated with greater pain intensity among patients with FM (45–47). Sayar et al. (47) compared levels of anger of patients with FM and RA. Even when severity of pain was controlled for, FM patients rated their anger as significantly higher than the RA patients. In particular, suppression of anger when experienced (anger-in) was significantly higher in the FM sample; however, anger-out (hostility and behavioral expression through verbal or physical means) coupled with anxiety explained 32% of the variance of pain severity reported by the FM patients. Despite also finding a high prevalence of anger in FM patients, Amir et al. (45) found no differences in the levels of anger reported by patients with FM, RA, and chronic low back pain.

Frustrations related to persistence of symptoms, limited information on etiology, and repeated treatment failures along with anger toward employers, insurance companies, the healthcare system, family members, and themselves, all contribute to the general dysphoric mood of patients (44). Kerns et al. (43) noted that internalization of angry feelings was strongly related to measures of pain intensity, perceived interference, and reported frequency of pain behaviors.

The precise mechanisms by which anger and frustration exacerbate pain are not known. One reasonable possibility is that anger exacerbates pain by increasing autonomic arousal (48). Anger may also block motivation for and acceptance of treatments oriented toward rehabilitation and disability management rather than cure. Yet rehabilitation and disability management are often the only treatments available for these patients.

In summary, it is important to be aware of the significant role of negative mood in FM because it is likely to influence treatment motivation and compliance with treatment recommendations. For example, patients who are anxious may fear engaging in what they perceive as demanding activities; patients who are depressed and who feel helpless may have little initiative to comply; and patients who are angry with the healthcare system are not likely to be motivated to respond to recommendations from yet another healthcare professional. Thus, clinicians who are treating people with FM must focus on their moods as well as physical pathology and somatic factors. Patients with FM cannot be treated successfully without attending to the patients' emotional state.

COGNITIVE FACTORS

As illustrated in the case of the butcher described by Tuke (1), people are not passive responders to physical sensation. Rather, they actively seek to make sense of their experience and respond based on their interpretation and not solely to objective information. They appraise their conditions by matching sensations to some preexisting implicit model and determine whether a particular sensation is a symptom of a particular physical disorder that requires attention or can be ignored. In this way, to some extent, each person functions with a uniquely constructed reality. When information is ambiguous, people rely on general attitudes and beliefs based on experience and prior learning history. These beliefs determine the meaning and significance of the problems, as well as the perceptions of appropriate treatment. If we accept the premise that pain is a complex, subjective phenomenon that is uniquely experienced by each person, then knowledge about idiosyncratic beliefs, appraisals, and coping repertoires becomes critical for optimal treatment planning and for accurately evaluating treatment outcome.

A great deal of research has been directed toward identifying cognitive factors that contribute to pain and disability (49,50). These studies have consistently demonstrated that patients' attitudes, beliefs, and expectancies about their plight, themselves, their coping resources, and their healthcare system affect their reports of pain, activity, disability, and response to treatment (51–53). The nature of important cognitive determinants of experience of behavior is worthy of exploration.

Beliefs About Pain

Clinicians working with chronic pain patients are aware that patients having similar pain histories and reports of pain may differ greatly in their beliefs about their pain. Certain beliefs may lead to maladaptive coping, exacerbation of pain, increased suffering, and greater disability. For example, if pain is interpreted as signifying ongoing tissue damage rather than being viewed as the result of a stable problem that may improve, it is likely to produce considerably more suffering and behavioral dysfunction even though the amount of nociceptive input in the two cases may be equivalent (54). People who believe that their pain is likely to persist may be quite passive in their coping efforts and fail to use cognitive or behavioral strategies to cope with pain. People with chronic pain who consider their pain as an unexplainable mystery may minimize their own abilities to control or decrease pain, and be less likely to rate their coping strategies as effective in controlling and decreasing pain (55,56).

Moreover for people with chronic pains' beliefs about the implications of a disease can affect their perception of symptoms. For example, Cassell (57) cited the case of a patient whose pain could easily be controlled with codeine when he attributed it to sciatica, but required significantly greater amounts of opioids to achieve the same degree of relief when he attributed it to metastatic cancer. Cassell's observation was confirmed in a study published by Spiegel and Bloom (54) who found that the pain severity ratings of cancer patients could be predicted not only by the use of analgesics and by the patients' affective state, but also by their *interpretations of pain*. Patients who attributed their pain to a worsening of their underlying disease experienced more pain than did patients with more benign interpretations, despite the same level of disease progression. These findings are reminiscent of the observation of Tuke's (1) butcher who reported great agony when he *thought* he had injured his arm, as described earlier.

A person's cognitions (beliefs, appraisals, expectancies) regarding the consequences of an event and his or her ability to deal with it are hypothesized to affect functioning in two ways—by directly influencing mood and indirectly influencing coping efforts. Both influences may affect physiological activity associated with pain such as muscle tension (58) and production of neuro-transmitters and endogenous opioids (59,60).

Most recently, there has been a shift in focus from patients' negative perceptions about their pain, to their healthcare providers' beliefs. Linton et al. (61) evaluated beliefs of healthcare providers regarding chronic pain, and reported that two-thirds of healthcare providers reported they would advise avoidance of pain-inducing activities, and more than 25% reported the belief that sick leave was beneficial in the recuperation from back pain. Further, patients who were recommended bed rest and analgesics as needed experienced more disability at follow-up as compared to patients who were recommended self-care strategies (11). This interaction among providers and patients high-lights the importance of social factors in pain experience.

The results of several studies suggest that when successful rehabilitation occurs, there appears to be an important cognitive shift—a shift from beliefs about helplessness and passivity to resourcefulness and ability to function regardless of pain. For example, Williams and Thorn (56) found that chronic pain patients who believed that their pain was an "unexplained mystery" reported high levels of psychological distress and pain, and also showed poorer treatment compliance than patients who believed that they understood their pain.

In a process study designed to evaluate the direct association between beliefs and symptoms of patients, a thought-sampling procedure was used to evaluate the nature of patients' cognitions during and immediately following headache, both prior to and following the treatment (62). Results indicated that there were significant changes in certain aspects of headache-related thinking in treated groups compared to a control group. Treated patients made significantly fewer negative appraisals (e.g., "It's getting worse," "There is nothing I can do") and significantly more positive appraisals than untreated patients. Treated patients learned to evaluate headaches in a more positive fashion. Importantly, patients who had the largest positive shifts in appraisal reported the greatest reduction in headache intensity. Remarkably, treated patients also reported significantly fewer headache days per week and lower intensity of pain than untreated controls.

Clearly, it appears essential for people with chronic pain to develop adaptive beliefs about the relation among impairment, pain, suffering, and disability, and to deemphasize the role of experienced pain in their regulation of functioning. In fact, results from numerous treatment outcome studies have shown that changes in pain level do not parallel changes in other variables of interest, including activity level, medication use, return to work, rated ability to cope with pain, and pursuit of further treatment (63,64).

Beliefs About Controllability

There are many laboratory studies demonstrating that controllability of aversive stimulation reduces its impact (65,66). Conversely, there is evidence that the explicit expectation of uncontrollable pain stimulation may cause subsequent nociceptive input to be perceived as more intense (67).

People with chronic pain typically perceive a lack of personal control, which probably relates to their ongoing but unsuccessful efforts to control their pain. A large proportion of chronic pain patients appear to believe that they have limited ability to exert control over their pain (50). Such negative, maladaptive appraisals about the situation and their personal efficacy may reinforce the experience of demoralization, inactivity, and overreaction to nociceptive stimulation commonly observed in chronic pain patients.

Self-Efficacy

Closely related to the sense of control over aversive stimulation is the concept of "self-efficacy." A self-efficacy expectation is defined as a personal conviction that one can successfully execute a course of action (i.e., perform required behaviors) to produce a desired outcome in a given situation. This construct appears to be a major mediator of therapeutic change.

Bandura (68,69) suggested that if a person has sufficient motivation to engage in a behavior, the person's self-efficacy beliefs are what determine which activities to initiate, the amount of effort expended, and extent of persistence in the face of obstacles and aversive experiences. Efficacy judgments are based on the following: (*i*) one's own past performance at the task or similar tasks, (*ii*) the performance accomplishments of others who are perceived to be similar to oneself, (*iii*) verbal persuasion by others that one is capable, and (*iv*) perception of one's own state of physiological arousal, which is in turn partly determined by prior efficacy estimation.

Lower self-efficacy beliefs, in particular, have been shown to be related to greater pain, disability, and depressive mood in FM (50,70). FM patients with lower self-efficacy who underwent a six-week training intervention involving physical training and exercise had lower posttreatment physical activity when compared to those with higher self-efficacy. Furthermore, improvements in self-efficacy during treatment were associated with lower tender point scores and pain intensity (70).

Encouraging patients to undertake subtasks that are increasingly difficult, or close to the desired behavioral repertoire, can create performance mastery experience. From this perspective, the occurrence of coping behaviors is conceptualized as being mediated by the individual's beliefs that situational demands do not exceed his or her coping resources.

Catastrophizing

Catastrophizing refers to extremely negative interpretations of one's circumstances and the future. Catastrophizing appears to greatly influence pain and disability (71,72). Following treatment, reductions in catastrophizing have been related to reduction in pain intensity and physical impairment. Flor and Turk (51) found that in low back pain patients and people with RA, significant percentages of the variance in pain and disability were accounted for by cognitive factors that were labeled as catastrophizing, helplessness, adaptive coping, and resourcefulness. In both the low back pain and the RA groups, the cognitive variables of catastrophizing and adaptive coping had substantially more explanatory power than did disease-related variables or impairment. Consistent results were reported by Keefe et al. (73) who found that RA patients who reported high levels of pain, physical disability, and depression had reported excessive catastrophizing ideation on questionnaires administered six months earlier.

In an effort to explore the combined predictive capacity of catastrophizing measures and physiological measures, Wolff and colleagues (74) evaluated lower paraspinal muscle tension and cardiac reactivity to emotional arousal, and found that high catastrophizers who had high resting muscle tension reported the highest pain levels. Additionally, high catastrophizers with low cardiovascular reactivity to emotional arousal reported the greatest pain levels. This experiment highlights the important interaction among physiological and cognitive factors in pain experience.

Coping
Self-regulation of pain and its impact depend on peoples' specific ways of dealing with pain, adjusting to pain, and reducing or minimizing distress caused by pain—in other words, their coping strategies. Coping is assumed to involve spontaneously employed, purposeful, and intentional acts, and it can be assessed in terms of overt and covert behaviors. Overt behavioral coping strategies include rest, use of relaxation techniques, or medication. Covert coping strategies include various means of distracting oneself from pain, reassuring oneself that the pain will diminish, seeking information, and problem-solving. Coping strategies likely act to alter both the perception of pain intensity and the ability to manage or tolerate pain and to continue everyday activities.

Studies have found active coping strategies (efforts to function in spite of pain or to distract oneself from pain, such as engaging in activity or ignoring pain) to be associated with adaptive functioning, and passive coping strategies (such as depending on others for help in pain control and restricting one's activities) to be related to greater pain and depression (53,75).

A number of studies have demonstrated that if individuals are instructed about the use of adaptive coping strategies, their ratings of pain intensity decrease and tolerance for pain increases (76). The most important factor in poor coping appears to be the presence of catastrophizing, rather than differences in the nature of specific adaptive coping strategies (77). Turk et al. (78) concluded that "what appears to distinguish low from high pain tolerant individuals are their cognitive processing, catastrophizing thoughts and feelings that precede, accompany, and follow aversive stimulation" (p. 197).

Hypervigilance
The diffused and generalized nature of FM has led some investigators to consider impairment or dysfunction in information processing as a critical factor in FM. The hypervigilance model for chronic pain suggests that some patients may be more sensitive to pain signals as a result of increased attention to somatosensory stimuli. Research investigating sensory processing of FM patients has consistently demonstrated that people with FM exhibit lower pain threshold than do age-matched and sex-matched healthy people (79,80). On the basis of

these results, Rollman and Lautenbacher (81) proposed a "hypervigilance model" in which heightened sensory vigilance is a predisposing factor in FM. Furthermore, vigilance to sensory information in FM may not be limited to pain. Some data indicate that FM patients are more sensitive to cold, noise, and environmental irritants (80,82), and a recent path analysis indicates that physical function impairment is mediated through comorbid physical symptoms (e.g., dizziness, shortness of breath) as a result of this sensory amplification (83).

PATIENT HETEROGENEITY

Although all of the psychosocial factors discussed are important to understanding the FM experience as a whole, it is equally important to understand that not all factors play an equivalent role for each individual with FM. A number of investigators have suggested that FM patients may not be a homogeneous group. Rather, there may be subgroups of people with FM. Studies have focused on differences depending on symptom onset, for example, idiopathic versus traumatic (84–86), symptom presentation (87), and psychological distress (88). The authors argue that delineation of the relevant subgroups will facilitate identification of the mechanisms underlying the symptoms of FM and the development of treatments customized to address specific needs of different patient groups.

Subgroups of FM patients have been identified based on a variety of psychosocial and behavioral factors (85,89,90). Schoenfeld-Smith et al. (90) performed a cluster analysis based on level of disability. They found that the best discriminator of the two resulting subgroups was perceived levels of helplessness. The group with poorer health status reported greater passive coping, helplessness and stress, and less satisfaction than the subgroup with better health status. Giesecke et al. (89) also identified subgroups of FM patients by looking at their mood, catastrophizing, perceived control, and muscle tenderness. These investigators found a subgroup with higher levels of emotional distress, catastrophizing, perceived control, and tenderness and a second subgroup with moderate levels of all of the psychological measures but low levels of tenderness. A third small subgroup was characterized by low levels of distress, high levels of perceived control, and extreme tenderness.

Turk and Rudy (91) developed an empirically derived taxonomy of chronic pain patients based upon patients' responses to the West Haven-Yale Multidimensional Pain Inventory (92) (MPI)—Dysfunctional (DYS), Interpersonally Distressed (ID), and Adaptive Copers (AC). The characteristics of these three subgroups are described in Table 3. The MPI comprises 12 subscales (i.e., pain,

TABLE 3 Characteristics of Chronic Pain Subgroups Based on MPI Profiles

Dysfunctional (DYS)	Interpersonally Distressed (ID)	Adaptive Copers (AC)
• Higher levels of pain • Higher levels of perceived interference with life • Higher levels of emotional distress • Lower levels of perceived control • Lower levels of activity	• Lower levels of perceived support • Higher levels of negative responses • Lower levels of solicitous responses • Lower levels of distracting responses	• Lower levels of pain • Lower levels of perceived interference • Lower levels of emotional distress • Higher levels of perceived control • Higher levels of activity

affective distress, perceived control, support, symptom interference, solicitous, distracting, and negative responses by significant others, and four subscales assessing different common physical activities). DYS patients are characterized by high levels of pain and emotional distress and low levels of perceived control and activity; ID patients by moderate levels of pain but low levels of support from significant others and high levels of negative responses from significant others; AC patients report relatively low levels of pain, mood, and activity interference and high levels of perceived control and general activity. There are some commonalities among these three efforts to identify patient subgroups based on psychosocial and behavioral factors. Since the greatest amount of work examining subgroups of chronic pain patients based on psychosocial and behavioral factors has been conducted by Turk and his colleagues, we will examine their subgroups in more detail.

The results of the Turk et al. (85) subgrouping study indicate that the majority of the FM patients (87%) can be classified into one of the three primary groups—DYS, ID, and AC—that have been previously identified for diverse chronic pain populations (92–94). The three FM groups differed significantly in opioid use, depression, pain severity, perceived disability, and level of marital satisfaction. Such differences were observed even though the groups exhibited comparable degrees of physical pathology and levels of physical functioning. The results revealed that the patients in the DYS group reported higher level of pain severity and opioid use than the ID and AC groups. The ID and DYS groups also differed significantly from the AC group in depression. The extent of marital satisfaction differentiated the two groups, with the ID patients reporting significantly lower level of satisfaction in their marriage than the DYS patients.

The distinct characteristics associated with each patient subgroup suggest that prescription of a uniformed intervention for all patients might result in less than optimal outcomes since the specific needs of some patients will not be directly addressed. It may be more appropriate to customize treatment in order to meet their specific clinical needs (95). For example, although the patients in both DYS and ID groups were depressed, depression in the latter group may be closely related to marital and interpersonal problems. Meaningful improvement, therefore, may not be achieved without addressing interpersonal or marital issues for ID FM patients. Being able to prescribe specific treatments based upon patient characteristics, rather than the more typical one-size-fits-all approach, is likely to benefit a greater number of patients and ultimately be more cost-effective. The value of customizing treatment to the three subgroups identified has been demonstrated in a growing number of studies (96,97).

Subgroups have also been identified based on patterns of symptom reporting. Recently we performed a cluster analysis on the symptom endorsement of FM participants in the online survey (87). Symptoms were grouped into three sets—(*i*) musculoskeletal symptoms (MS) of FM (e.g., pain, stiffness), (*ii*) nonmusculoskeletal (NMS) physical symptoms (e.g., rashes, abdominal pain), and (*iii*) cognitive and psychological (CP) symptoms (e.g., anxiety, forgetfulness)—and then performed a cluster analysis of these sets of symptoms. One group was characterized by high scores on all three sets of symptoms and a second with low scores on all symptoms. Two additional groups were also discovered. One had moderate scores on both physical symptoms but low scores on the CP symptoms. The final subgroup also had moderate scores on the physical symptoms but high scores on the CP symptoms. These data indicate that FM patients differ substantially in the types of symptoms they report. The data also demonstrate that only one-half of the patients report severe problems with CP symptoms. Whether the failure to acknowledge the CP symptoms results from denial or is an accurate reflection is unknown. These results, however, have important implications for treatment as they suggest that different treatments may be indicated based on the types of symptoms present.

To summarize, it is important to acknowledge that FM patients are not a homogeneous group (83). It is reasonable to assume that large individual differences existed prior to the development of FM and that these differences persist or are magnified in response to the stress associated with a chronic condition. Thus, although the evolving processes may be present in all FM patients, the degrees to which the processes become dysregulated may vary across people due to differences in the predispositional factors (98). Subgroups may respond to an identical intervention in different manners. Consequently, the "one-size-fits-all" approach of treating FM patients is not likely to be effective. Identification of patients' characteristics and matching them to specific treatment may be needed to maximize clinical efficacy.

SUMMARY AND CONCLUSIONS

The variability of patients' responses to nociceptive stimuli and treatment is somewhat more understandable when we consider that pain is a personal experience influenced by attention, meaning of the situation, and prior learning history as well as physical pathology. In the majority of cases, biomedical factors appear to instigate the initial report of pain. Over time, however, secondary problems associated with deconditioning may exacerbate and serve to maintain the problem. Inactivity leads to increased focus on and preoccupation with the body and pain, and these cognitive-attentional changes increase the likelihood of misinterpreting symptoms, the overemphasis on symptoms, and the patient's self-perception as disabled. Reduction of activity, anger, fear of reinjury, pain, loss of compensation, and an environment that perhaps unwittingly supports the *pain patient role* can impede alleviation of pain, successful rehabilitation, reduction of disability, and improvement in adjustment.

Pain that persists over time should not be viewed as either solely physical or solely psychological. Rather, the experience of pain is a complex amalgam maintained by an interdependent set of biomedical, psychosocial, and behavioral factors, whose relationships are not static but evolve and change over time. The various interacting factors that affect a person with chronic pain suggest that the phenomenon is quite complex and requires a biopsychosocial perspective.

From the biopsychosocial perspective, each of these factors contributes to the experience of pain and the response to treatment. The interaction among the various factors is what produces the subjective experience of pain. There is a synergistic relationship whereby psychological and socio-environmental factors can modulate nociceptive stimulation and the response to treatment. In turn, nociceptive stimulation can influence patients' appraisals of their situation and the treatment, their mood states, and the ways they interact with significant others, including medical practitioners. An integrative, biopsychosocial model of chronic pain needs to incorporate the mutual interrelationships among physical, psychological, and social factors and the changes that occur among these relationships over time (99,100). The treatment approach that focuses on only one of these three core sets of factors will inevitably be incomplete.

ACKNOWLEDGMENT
Support for the preparation of this manuscript was provided in part from a grant from the National Institutes of Health, NIAMS grant # AR 44724.

REFERENCES
1. Tuke DH. Illustrations of the Influence of the Mind Upon the Body in Health and Disease Designed to Elucidate the Imagination. 2nd ed. Philadelphia: Henry C. Lea, 1884.
2. Hudson JI, Pope HG Jr. The relationship between fibromyalgia and major depressive disorder. Rheum Dis Clin North Am 1996; 22:285–303.
3. Arnold LM, Hudson JI, Hess EV, et al. Family study of fibromyalgia. Arthritis Rheum 2004; 50:944–952.
4. Arnold LM, Hudson JI, Keck PE, et al. Comorbidity of fibromyalgia and psychiatric disorders. J Clin Psychiatry 2006; 67:1219–1225.
5. Goldenberg DL. Fibromyalgia syndrome a decade later: what have we learned? Arch Intern Med 1999; 159:777–785.
6. White KP, Nielson WR, Harth M, et al. Chronic widespread musculoskeletal pain with or without fibromyalgia: psychological distress in a representative community adult sample. J Rheumatol 2002; 29:588–594.
7. Bennett RM, Jones J, Turk DC, et al. An internet survey of 2,596 people with fibromyalgia. BMC Musculoskeletal Dis 2007; 8:27.
8. Carey M, Burish T. Etiology and treatment of the psychological side effects associated with cancer chemotherapy: a critical review and discussion. Psychol Bull 1988; 104:307–325.
9. Fordyce W. Behavioral Methods in Chronic Pain and Illness. St. Louis: CV Mosby, 1976.
10. Turk DC, Okifuji A. Perception of traumatic onset and compensation status: impact on pain severity, emotional distress, and disability in chronic pain patients. J Behav Med 1996; 9:435–453.
11. Von Korff M, Barlow W, Cherkin D, et al. The effects of practice style in managing back pain. Ann Intern Med 1994; 121:182–195.
12. Thieme K, Flor H, Turk DC. Psychological treatment in fibromyalgia syndrome: efficacy of operant behavioural and cognitive behavioural treatments. Arthritis Res Ther 2006; 8:R121.Available at: http://arthritis-reseach-com/content/8/4/R121.
13. Thieme K, Gromnica-Ihle E, Flor H. Operant behavioral treatment of fibromyalgia: a controlled study. Arthritis Rheum 2003; 49:314–320.
14. Merskey H, Bogduk N. Classification of chronic pain. Descriptions of chronic pain syndromes and definitions of pain terms. Pain 1986: S1–226.
15. Fernandez E. Anxiety, Depression, and Anger in Pain: Research Implications. Dallas, TX: Advanced Psychology Resources, 2002.
16. Wolfe F, Smythe HA, Yunus MB, et al. The American College of Rheumatology 1990 criteria for the classification of fibromyalgia: report of the multicenter criteria committee. Arthritis Rheum 1990; 36:160–172.
17. Berger A, Dukes E, Martin S, et al. Characteristics and healthcare costs of patients with fibromyalgia syndrome. Int J Clin Pract 2007; 61:1498–1508.
18. Vlaeyen JWS, Kole-Snijders AM, Boeren RGB, et al. Fear of movement/(re)injury in chronic low back pain and its relation to behavioral performance. Pain 1995; 62:363–372.
19. Vlaeyen JWS, Linton SJ. Fear-avoidance and its consequences in chronic musculoskeletal pain: a state of the art. Pain 2000; 85:317–332.
20. Vlaeyen JWS, Seelen HAM, Peters M, et al. Fear of movement/(re)injury and muscular reactivity in chronic low back pain patients: an experimental investigation. Pain 1999; 82:297–304.

21. Bayer T, Baer PE, Early C. Situational and psychophysiolgical factors in psychologically induced pain. Pain 1991; 44:45–50.
22. Lenthem J, Slade PD, Troup JDG, et al. Outline of a fear-avoidance model of exaggerated pain perception—I. Behav Res Ther 1983; 21:401–408.
23. McCracken LM, Gross RT, Sorg PJ, et al. Prediction of pain in patients with chronic low back pain: effects of inaccurate prediction and pain-related anxiety. Behav Res Ther 1993; 31:647–652.
24. Aghabeigi B, Feinmann C, Harris M. Prevalence of post-traumatic stress disorder in patients with chronic idiopathic facial pain. Br J Oral Maxillofacial Surg 1992; 30:360–364.
25. Amital D, Fostick L, Polliack ML, et al. Posttraumatic stress disorder, tenderness, and fibromyalgia syndrome: are they different entities? J Psychosomat Res 2006; 61:663–669.
26. Cohen J, Neumann L, Haiman Y, et al. Prevalence of post-traumatic stress disorder in fibromyalgia patients: overlapping syndromes or post-traumatic fibromyalgia syndrome? Semin Arthritis Rheum 2002; 32:38–50.
27. Sherman JJ, Turk DC, Okifuji A. Prevalence and impact of posttraumatic stress disorder (PTSD) symptoms on patients with fibromyalgia syndrome. Clin J Pain 2000; 16:127–134.
28. Raphael KG, Janal MN, Nayak S, et al. Psychiatric comorbidities in a community sample of women with fibromyalgia. Pain 2006; 124:117–125.
29. First M, Spitzer R, Gibbon M, et al. Structured Clinical Interview for DSM-IV Axis I Disorders—Nonpatient Edition. New York, NY: Biometrics Research Department, New York Psychiatric Institute, 1995.
30. Banks SM, Kerns RD. Explaining high rates of depression in chronic pain: a diathesis-stress framework. Psychol Bull 1996; 119:95–110.
31. Wolfe F, Ross K, Anderson J, et al. The prevalence and characteristics of fibromyalgia in the general population. Arthritis Rheum 1995; 38:19–28.
32. Atkinson JH, Slater MA, Patterson TL, et al. Prevalence, onset, and risk of psychiatric disorders in men with chronic low back pain: a controlled study. Pain 1991; 45:111–121.
33. Magni G, Moreschi C, Rigatti Luchini S, et al. Prospective study on the relationship between depressive symptoms and chronic musculoskeletal pain. Pain 1994; 56:289–297.
34. Rudy TE, Kerns RD, Turk DC. Chronic pain and depression: toward a cognitive-behavioral mediation model. Pain 1988; 35:129–140.
35. Brown GK. A causal analysis of chronic pain and depression. J Abnorm Psychol 1990; 99:127–137.
36. Katon W, Egan K, Miller D. Chronic pain: lifetime psychiatric diagnoses and family history. Am J Psychiatry 1985; 142:1156–1160.
37. Jarvik JG, Hollingworth W, Heagerty PJ, et al. Three-year incidence of low back pain in an initially asymptomatic cohort. clinical and imaging risk factors. Spine 2005; 30:1541–1548.
38. Von Korff M, Simon G. The relationship between pain and depression. Brit J Psychiatry 1996; 168(suppl 30):101–108.
39. Robinson RL, Birnbaum HG, Morley MA, et al. Depression and fibromyalgia: treatment and cost when diagnosed separately or currently. J Rheumatol 2004; 31:1621–1629.
40. Fernandez E, Turk DC. The scope and significant of anger in the experience of chronic pain. Pain 1995; 61:165–175.
41. Schwartz L, Slater M, Birchler G, et al. Depression in spouses of chronic pain patients: the role of patient pain and anger, and marital satisfaction. Pain 1991; 44:61–67.
42. Greenwood KA, Thurston R, Rumble M, et al. Anger and persistent pain: current status and future directions. Pain 2003; 103:1–5.
43. Kerns RD, Rosenberg R, Jacob MC. Anger expression and chronic pain. J Behav Med 1994; 17:57–68.

44. Okifuji A, Turk DC, Curran SL. Anger in chronic pain: investigations of anger targets and intensity. J Psychosom Res 1999; 61:771–780.
45. Amir M, Neumann L, Bor O, et al. Coping styles, anger social support, and suicide risk of women with fibromyalgia syndrome. J Musculoskel Pain 2000; 8:7–20.
46. Conant LL. Psychological variables associated with pin perceptions among individuals with chronic spinal cord injury pain. J Clin Psychol Med Settings 1998; 5:71–90.
47. Sayar K, Gulec H, Topbas M. Alexthymia and anger in patients with fibromyalgia. Clin Rheumatol 2004; 23:441–448.
48. Burns JW. Anger management style and hostility: predicting symptom-specific physiological reactivity among chronic low back pain patients. J Behav Med 1997; 20:505–522.
49. Jensen MP, Turner JA, Romano JM, et al. Coping with chronic pain: a critical review of the literature. Pain 1991; 47:249–283.
50. Turk DC, Okifuji A. Psychological factors in chronic pain: evolution and revolutions. J Consult Clin Psychol 2002; 70:678–690.
51. Flor H, Turk DC. Chronic back pain and rheumatoid arthritis: predicting pain and disability from cognitive variables. J Behav Med 1988; 11:51–265.
52. Jensen MP, Turner JA, Romano JM, et al. Relationship of pain-specific beliefs to chronic pain adjustment. Pain 1994; 57:301–309.
53. Tota-Faucette ME, Gil KM, Keefe FJ, et al. Predictors of response to pain management treatment. The role of family environment and changes in cognitive processes. Clin J Pain 1993; 9:115–123.
54. Spiegel D, Bloom JR. Pain in metastatic breast cancer. Cancer 1983; 52:341–345.
55. Williams DA, Keefe FJ. Pain beliefs and the use of cognitive-behavioral coping strategies. Pain 1991; 46:185–190.
56. Williams DA, Thorn BE. An empirical assessment of pain beliefs. Pain 1989; 36:251–258.
57. Cassell EJ. The nature of suffering and the goals of medicine. N Engl J Med 1982; 396:639–645.
58. Flor H, Turk DC, Birbaumer N. Assessment of stress-related psychophysiological responses in chronic pain patients. J Consult Clin Psychol 1985; 35:354–364.
59. Bandura A, O'Leary A, Taylor CB, et al. Perceived self-efficacy and pain control: opioid and nonopioid mechanisms. J Pers Soc Psychol 1987; 53:563–571.
60. Bandura A, Taylor CB, Williams SL, et al. Catecholamine secretion as a function of perceived coping self-efficacy. J Consult Clin Psychol 1985; 53:406–414.
61. Linton SJ, Vlaeyen JW, Ostello RW. The back pain beliefs of health care providers: are we fear-avoidant? J Occup Rehabil 2002; 12:223–232.
62. Newton CR, Barbaree HE. Cognitive changes accompanying headache treatment: the use of a thought-sampling procedure. Cogn Ther Res 1987; 11:635–652.
63. Flor H, Fydrich T, Turk DC. Efficacy of multidisciplinary pain treatment centers: a meta-analytic review. Pain 1992; 49:221–230.
64. Jensen MP, Karoly P. Control beliefs, coping effort, and adjustment to chronic pain. J Consult Clin Psychol 1991; 59:431–438.
65. Morley S, Eccleston C, Williams A. Systematic review and meta-analysis of randomized controlled trials of cognitive behaviour therapy and behaviour therapy for chronic pain in adults, excluding headache. Pain 1999; 80:1–13.
66. Wells N. Perceived control over pain: relation to distress and disability. Res Nurs Health 1994; 17:295–302.
67. Leventhal H, Everhart D. Emotion, pain and physical Illness. In: Izard CE, ed. Emotion and Psychopathology. New York: Plenum Press, 1979:263–299.
68. Bandura A. Self-efficacy: toward a unifying theory of behavioral change. Psychol Rev 1977; 84:191–215.
69. Bandura A. Self-efficacy. The Exercise of Control. New York: W.H. Freeman, 1997.
70. Buckelew, SP, Murray SE, Hewett JE, et al. Self-efficacy, pain, and physical activity among fibromyalgia subjects. Arthritis Care Res 1995; 8:43–50.
71. Keefe FJ, Caldwell DS, Williams DA, et al. Pain coping skills training in the management of osteoarthritis knee pain: a comparative approach. Behav Ther 1990; 21:49–62.

72. Keefe FJ, Caldwell DS, Williams DA, et al. Pain coping skills training in the management of osteoarthritis knee pain II. Follow-up results. Behav Ther 1990; 21:435–447.
73. Keefe FJ, Brown GK, Wallston KS, et al. Coping with rheumatoid arthritis pain. Catastrophizing as a maladaptive strategy. Pain 1989; 37:51–56.
74. Wolff B, Burns JW, Quartana PJ, et al. Pain catastrophizing, physiological indexes, and chronic pain severity: tests of mediation and moderations models. J Behav Med 2008; 31:105–114.
75. Lawson K, Reesor KA, Keefe FJ, et al. Dimensions of pain–related cognitive coping: cross–validation of the factor structure of the Coping Strategy Questionnaire. Pain 1990; 43:195–204.
76. Fernandez E, Turk DC. The utility of cognitive coping strategies for altering perception of pain: a meta-analysis. Pain 1989; 38:123–135.
77. Heyneman NE, Fremouw WJ, Gano D, et al. Individual differences in the effectiveness of different coping strategies. Cogn Ther Res 1990; 14:63–77.
78. Turk DC, Meichenbaum D, Genest M. Pain and Behavioral Medicine: A Cognitive-Behavioral Perspective. New York: Guilford Press, 1983.
79. Kosek E, Ekholm J, Hansson P. Sensory dysfunction in fibromyalgia patients with implications for pathogenic mechanisms. Pain 1996; 68:375–383.
80. McDermid AJ, Rollman GB, McCain GA. Generalized hypervigilance in fibromyalgia: evidence of perceptual amplification. Pain 1996; 66:133–144.
81. Rollman GB, Lautenbacher S. Hypervigilance effects in fibromyalgia: pain experience and pain perception. In: Værøy H, Merskey H, eds. Progress in Fibromyalgia and Myofascial Pain. Amsterdam: Elsevier, 1993.
82. Nørregaard J, Bülow PM, Mehlsen J, et al. Biochemical changes in relation to a maximal exercise test in patients with fibromyalgia. Clin Physiol 1994; 14:159–167.
83. Geisser ME, Donnell CS, Petzke F, et al. Comorbid somatic symptoms and functional status in patients with fibromyalgia and chronic fatigue syndrome: sensory amplification as a common mechanism. Psychosomatics 2008; 49:235–242.
84. Greenfield S, Fitzcharles MA, Esdaile JM. Reactive fibromyalgia syndrome. Arthritis Rheum 1992; 35:678–681.
85. Turk DC, Okifuji A, Sinclair JD, et al. Pain, disability, and physical functioning in subgroups of patients with fibromyalgia. J Rheum 1996; 23:1255–1262.
86. Waylonis GW, Perkins RH. Post-traumatic fibromyalgia. A long-term follow-up. Am J Phys Med Rehabil 1994; 73:403–412.
87. Wilson HD, Robinson JP, Turk DC. Toward the identification of symptom patterns in people with fibromyalgia. Arthritis Rheum 2009; 61(4):527–534.
88. Turk DC, Flor H. Primary fibromyalgia greater than tender points: toward a multiaxial taxonomy. J Rheumatol 1989; 16:80–86.
89. Giesecke T, Williams DA, Harris RE, et al. Subgroups of fibromyalgia patients on the basis of pressure-pain thresholds and psychological factors. Arthritis Rheum 2003; 48:2916–2922.
90. Schoenfeld-Smith K, Nicassio PM, Radojevic V, et al. Multiaxial taxonomy of fibromyalgia syndrome patients. J Clin Psychol Med Settings 1995; 2:149–166.
91. Kerns RD, Turk DC, Rudy TE. The West Haven-Yale Multidimensional Pain Inventory (WHYMPI). Pain 1985; 23:345–356.
92. Turk DC, Rudy TE. Toward an empirically derived taxonomy of chronic pain states: a integration of psychological assessment data. J Consult Clin Psychol 1988; 56:233–238.
93. Turk DC, Rudy TE. The robustness of an empirically derived taxonomy of chronic pain patients. Pain 1990; 42:27–35.
94. Turk DC, Sist TC, Okifuji A, et al. Adaptation to metastatic cancer pain, regional/local cancer pain and non-cancer pain: role of psychological and behavioral factors. Pain 1998; 74:247–256.
95. Turk DC. Customizing treatment for chronic pain patients: who, what, and why. Clin J Pain 1990; 6:255–270.
96. Bergstrom G, Jensen IB, Bodin L, et al. The impact of psychologically different patient groups on outcome after a vocational rehabilitation program for long-term spinal pain patients. Pain 2001; 93:229–237.

97. Talo S, Forssell H, Heikkonen S, et al. Integrative group therapy outcome related to psychosocial characteristics in patients with chronic pain. Int J Rehabil Res 2001; 24:25–33.
98. Okifuji A, Turk D. Fibromyalgia: search for mechanisms and effective treatments. In: Gatchel RJ, Turk DC, eds. Psychological Factors in Pain: Evolution and Revolution. New York: Guilford, 1999:227–246.
99. Flor H, Birbaumer N, Turk DC. The psychobiology of chronic pain. Adv Behav Res Ther 1990; 12:47–84.
100. Turk DC, Monarch ES. Biopsychosocial perspective on pain. In: Turk DC, Gatchel RJ, eds. Psychological Approaches to Pain Management: A Practitioner's Handbook. 2nd ed. New York: Guilford Press, 2002:3–39.

6 Disability Management in Patients with Fibromyalgia Syndrome

Raymond C. Tait and Vikrum Figoora
Department of Neurology and Psychiatry, Saint Louis University School of Medicine, St. Louis, Missouri, U.S.A.

INTRODUCTION

The fibromyalgia syndrome (FMS) is widespread, representing the second, most common disorder seen by rheumatologists and affecting between 2% and 4% of the U.S. adult population (1,2). Prevalence estimates vary in part because of some uncertainty in criteria used to diagnose the condition, despite the widespread acceptance of criteria promulgated by the American College of Rheumatology (ACR) almost 20 years ago (3). In part, estimates vary because FMS commonly co-occurs with other health conditions, further complicating its diagnosis (4). While there can be multiple precipitants for FMS and its mechanisms remain unclear (5), there is increasing evidence that FMS reflects a disorder of central nervous system processing, rather than abnormalities of muscle or other soft tissues (6–8). Although the specific mechanisms remain unclear, there now is a general agreement that it is a bona fide diagnostic entity, generally characterized by the ACR criteria.

A constellation of symptoms characterizes FMS. Its diagnosis requires the presence of widespread pain and mild or greater tenderness on palpation of at least 11 of 18 preidentified tender points (ACR). That said, the severity of symptoms can wax and wane, such that a person who demonstrates multiple trigger points at one point in time may exhibit fewer at another. Despite this variation in symptom severity, the latter patient generally would meet criteria for diagnosis (9,10). Aside from widespread pain, other symptoms commonly occur and include fatigue, sleep disturbance, headaches, and psychiatric comorbidities, especially depression and anxiety (11–13). Not surprisingly, FMS patients with this constellation of symptoms, especially those for whom symptom severity is high, also demonstrate significant functional interference and work disability (1,14–16).

Disability assessment and management, the foci of this chapter, are important in FMS patients for several reasons. Relative to management issues, there is evidence that effectively minimizing the disabling impact of pain can favorably impact a range of long-term clinical outcomes broadly associated with a patient's quality of life (17). Such management can be especially meaningful for FMS patients, for whom studies have shown a tendency for disability to progress over time (18,19). Moreover, recent research suggests some approaches to disability management that may reduce the likelihood of that progression (20–23), such that clinical improvement may be possible if these approaches are integrated into care.

Of course, despite progress in the treatment of FMS-related disability, a significant number of FMS patients will demonstrate functional decline over time, meaning that practitioners will face issues relative to disability evaluation in a significant minority of their patients. Because FMS patients often demonstrate few "objective" findings that can account for the severity of their symptoms and their levels of disability (15), disability evaluation can be challenging in the face of disability compensation paradigms that rely heavily on such findings. Though challenging, the practitioner is in the best position to assist in the disability determination process, so an understanding of factors that weigh in that process can be useful.

The following sections will address these issues, primarily focusing on perspectives of potential value to the practitioner who treats FMS patients. In the first section, we address basic considerations regarding definitions of disability, functional interference, and impairment. We also examine what is known about the disability trajectory in the general population of FMS patients and the factors known to contribute to disability in that group. The second section focuses on approaches to treatment relative to their impact on FMS-related disability. The third section addresses issues related to disability determination in FMS, with particular attention to prevailing paradigms that militate against accurate assessment of disability and to issues that practitioners should address as they evaluate levels of disability. The chapter concludes with a discussion of directions for future research that have promising possibilities for managing the disabling impact of FMS.

DISABILITY
Definitions

Several terms are often used and confused in discussions of pain-related disability, such as impairment. While impairment is a term that is defined variably depending on the agency offering the definition, all definitions center on limitations related to bodily functions and/or structures (24). For example, the World Health Organization defines impairments as either structural (anomaly, defect, loss) or functional problems that occasion significant deviation or loss. Similarly, the *American Medical Association Guides to the Evaluation of Permanent Impairment, 5th edition* (*AMA Guides 5th*) offers the following definition (25, p. 2): "A loss, loss of use, or derangement of any body part, organ system, or organ function." The definition offered by the Social Security Administration goes a step further, requiring that any such loss be verifiable by "medically acceptable" diagnostic techniques.

If impairment refers to limitations of organ structure or function, disability refers to limitations of activity secondary to an existing impairment. Thus, disability involves an inability to execute important daily tasks because of a medical condition or impairment. Recently, the concept of disability has been further refined into two components: functional limitations and participative limitations. Functional limitations refer to interference with abilities to carry out specific activities in daily life (e.g., climbing a flight of stairs, walking a mile). By comparison, participative limitations reference inabilities to carry out customary role functions (e.g., work, home). Obviously, functional and participative limitations are related, but the relationship is not isomorphic. A classic example involves a concert pianist with an injury to the little finger on his nondominant hand; while the injury limits only a small set of daily activities, these limitations are disabling relative to his role as a concert performer.

These and other considerations make assessing disability secondary to persistent pain a frustrating exercise for both healthcare providers and patients, not least because of the uncertain relationship between "objective findings" of impairment (as revealed, e. g., on MRI) and reports of pain and pain-related interference with life activities. The above problem applies not only to chronic pain conditions generally, but to the pain of FMS, specifically. The uncertainty, of course, is particularly problematic when the assessment relates to the determination of disability benefits, a determination that relies heavily on objective findings. (Issues specific to disability determination will be addressed at length in a later section of this chapter.)

The following sections will address factors that contribute to functional and role limitations in patients with FMS. We will use the terms functional limitations and functional interference interchangeably with the term disability throughout the chapter, except when specifically referencing occupational role limitations. The latter case will be referenced specifically as work disability. An understanding of factors associated with disability is useful for the practitioner interested in managing the component parts of FMS-related disability so as to minimize the overall impact of disability often endemic to the syndrome.

Disability in FMS

Abundant evidence attests to the disabling impact of FMS. A large multicenter study conducted in the United States reported that over 35% of FMS patients reported symptoms that were sufficiently severe that the patients missed substantial time from work, with 26.5% receiving some form of disability payment and 14.4% receiving Social Security Disability Insurance (SSDI) benefits (26). A smaller Canadian study reported similar results (1): 31% reported work disability and 26% reported receiving disability awards secondary to FMS. Of course, there is variation in rates of disability across studies: both lower rates (25% reporting disability, 15% receiving SSDI benefits) (27) and higher rates (46.8% reporting FMS-related job loss) (28) also have been reported. Notwithstanding some variability, these data show that FMS is consistently associated with high rates of disability. This association is further supported by several sources of national data: a study of disability awards in Norway showed FMS to be the most frequent diagnosis for people who received such awards in 1988 (29), and data from Canadian insurance carriers showed that FMS diagnoses accounted for 9% of their disability payments annually (30).

Not only is FMS-related disability widespread, it also has proved difficult to manage. As noted earlier, most studies show that FMS symptoms worsen or, at best, remain relatively stable over the course of time (18,19,31). Studies of the course of disability in FMS parallel those described above: levels of disability stay the same or worsen over the course of time, even when care is provided in specialty rheumatology clinics. For example, a longitudinal Norwegian study of 44 FMS patients found that the number receiving a full disability pension increased from 10 at baseline to 21 at follow-up 4.5 years later (32). Similarly, a large study involving multiple U.S. sites reported significant worsening of self-reported disability over the course of seven years (19), and a Canadian study also showed some deterioration in physical function and a significant increase in the percentage of patients claiming total disability over an 18-month period (33).

Although the latter data do not seem promising relative to their implications for the management of disability in FMS, it is important to recognize that many of the studies are relatively dated. Over the past decade, FMS has been recognized as a bona fide clinical condition, and our understanding has grown of central processing mechanisms associated with it. Indeed, there now are FDA-approved medications with indications for treating FMS, a relatively recent development (34,35), as well as evidence regarding nonpharmacological treatments with demonstrated effectiveness (20). Evidence also has accrued relative to factors that are associated with FMS-related disability, describing possible targets for further interventions for FMS. Before moving to the results of treatment studies, it is important to understand the factors that can contribute to disability in FMS: these factors often represent bona fide targets for treatment.

Factors Affecting FMS-Related Disability

As noted previously, considerable research has attempted, without success, to identify neuromuscular pathology that might explain FMS symptomatology, including FMS-related disability (14,36). In the absence of such evidence, numerous studies have examined other factors related to disability in FMS patients. While disability has been operationalized differently across studies (some examining self-reported functional limitations, others assessing actual physical performance, and others addressing work-related limitations), results have been reasonably consistent, such that the studies can be divided into four categories where relations between FMS and disability have been examined. First, we examine the evidence brought to bear on the assertion that the mere diagnosis of FMS can occasion disability. Then, we review the evidence-linking measures of physical symptoms (e.g., pain severity, tender points, fatigue) and FMS-related disability. This is followed by a review of the data examining environmental factors that may be related to work disability among FMS patients. Finally, we examine associations between psychological factors and FMS-related disability.

FMS Labeling

As with other painful conditions, concerns have been raised that the mere act of labeling a patient as having FMS may occasion increased disability. The arguments that link labeling and disability are well reasoned and generally note that such labels can produce anxiety and/or feelings of helplessness/resignation. Both of these reactions may augment medically unexplained symptoms or, at least, the patient's perceptions of the severity of those symptoms, and promote illness behavior (37–39). Given that FMS patients have been found to demonstrate disordered symptom appraisal (40) and generally enhanced sensitivity to various sensory stimuli (41), such arguments have presumptive merit.

Although this matter has been widely debated (6), relatively little empirical evidence is available on the matter. In one study that specifically examined this issue, 72 previously undiagnosed patients were identified as meeting the criteria for a diagnosis of FMS (33). The clinical status of these 72 patients was compared to that of 28 patients who had received prior FMS diagnoses; the previously diagnosed patients were significantly worse across virtually all metrics. The previously undiagnosed patients then were reassessed at 18 months (for 56 patients, 78% of the initial sample) and 36 months (for 43 patients, 60% of the initial sample) in order to evaluate the effect of labeling. Results showed increased symptomatology at 18 months and modest improvement relative to baseline at 36 months. There was, however, a nonsignificant self-reported decline in function at the 36-month mark and an increase in the number of patients reporting total disability (34.9% vs. 23.3% at baseline).

Although the above study involved a limited sample, the data do not show a profound impact of labeling on disability. That said, a substantial proportion of the original sample reported total disability by the end of the study, and a reasonable proportion developed disability over the 36-month study period, so the results do not close the door on this argument. Indeed, recent research has found discriminable clusters of FMS patients (42,43): (*i*) a subgroup characterized by low levels of tenderness and moderate levels of psychological distress/impaired coping, (*ii*) a subgroup characterized by high levels of tenderness and low levels of psychological distress/impaired coping, and (*iii*) a subgroup characterized by high levels of tenderness and high levels of psychological distress/impaired coping. Because patients in the latter group may be more vulnerable to phenomena such as labeling effects, the topic may merit further study.

Physical Symptoms

Physical symptoms such as the number of tender points, level of pain severity, and coexisting fatigue and/or weakness are associated with FMS-related disability. Not surprisingly, there is abundant evidence of an association between levels of pain severity and levels of disability, whether disability is assessed by self-report (10), by objective measures of performance (44–46), or by work absence/disability (1,47). Tender points (both tender point count and tender point sensitivity) also have demonstrated strongly positive relationships with self-report measures of activity interference and disability benefits (1,10). Interestingly, even though tender points are a cardinal feature of FMS that is required by ACR diagnosis and, heretofore, a useful inclusion criterion for research purposes, there is discussion that the tender points may be a less reliable indicator of clinical FMS than more global assessments (9). Indeed, strict reliance on the tender point criterion has been identified as a possible reason that FMS is more commonly diagnosed in women than men: men may report fewer tender points than women, even if they demonstrate all of the other symptoms typically required for the diagnosis.

Fatigue and weakness are common physical symptoms of FMS. As noted previously, pathophysiological studies have not yielded evidence of symptom causation. Despite the lack of evidence of a causal mechanism, research suggests that these symptoms contribute significantly to FMS-related disability. Indeed, in a study comparing women with FMS and age-matched (~46 years of age) and weight-matched controls against an older (~72 years of age) cohort of healthy women, FMS patients were more comparable to the older group than to the matched controls: their levels of lower extremity strength and general functionality were significantly lower than those of the latter group, but did not differ from those of the former group (14).

The physical deficits described above also have been demonstrated in studies of general ambulatory activity: relative to controls, FMS patients recorded low peak levels of activity and less time involved in high-level exertion (45). Such deficits in strength and endurance have been shown to contribute significantly to work-related disability, especially in the short term (47). Moreover, in the absence of job flexibility, these deficits can occasion long-term disability at levels that can impact job status (48). In fact, fatigue may contribute more to work disability than pain (48–50), possibly because it often co-occurs with persistent sleep disturbance and depression (51). Such results underscore the importance of viewing the physical symptoms associated with disability in conjunction with other variables known to impact functional status.

Environmental Factors and Disability
The literature regarding relations between the environment and work disability in FMS patients can be divided into three areas: (*i*) the occupational environment; (*ii*) the home environment; and (*iii*) the larger, socioeconomic environment. Although the empirical evidence in each area is limited, maximum attention has been paid to the occupational environment. Relative to the latter, evidence suggests that FMS patients, secondary to a constellation of symptoms (pain, fatigue, decreased muscle strength, limited endurance), demonstrate reduced work capacity. Whether FMS patients with reduced work capacity can remain in the workforce depends on several factors (49). One involves the absolute level of physical demands that FMS patients face in the workplace (52); this is a particularly significant factor in short-term, sick leaves (53). Other job-related factors, however, appear to mediate long-term absences from the workforce. A factor of particular importance involves a worker's job flexibility, the ability to vary work tasks, the pace of work, and/or the positions that must be maintained over the course of a work day (49,54). Another factor involves the emotional climate of the workplace, particularly the levels of coworker support and job satisfaction (53). Indeed, emotional factors may play an even larger role in long-term employment: FMS patients described significant emotional benefits from employment, as well as benefit from the structure that regular employment provides (48). It is noteworthy that many of the factors described above have been shown to influence employment over the long term for patients with other chronic pain conditions; therefore, these findings are relevant to the management of pain from any source in the setting of long-term employment (55).

While less studied, demands outside the workplace, particularly at home, also appear to influence long-term employment for women. Thus, working women who also have primary responsibility for the household (e.g., heavy household tasks, caring for small children) are at greater risk for leaving the workforce (54). Similar considerations apply to transportation to work: women with lengthy commutes describe such transportation issues as significant impediments to employment (48). Interestingly, domestic factors have not been studied in FMS-related disability among men.

Demographic and socioeconomic factors also have received sparse attention in studies of disability and FMS. Not surprisingly, those data indicate that socioeconomic factors, especially level of education, contribute to the likelihood of occupational disability (1,49). Similarly, demographic factors, including age at FMS onset, also can influence disability. While other socioeconomic (e.g., neighborhood, insurance status) and demographic factors (e.g., race, ethnicity) have not been studied explicitly in FMS patients relative to the likelihood of disability, there is reason to believe that associations exist in ways similar to those identified in other chronic pain groups (56). As discussed in the next section, the pattern of results is consistent with a diathesis-stress model of pain and disability (57).

Psychological Factors and Disability

Psychological factors have been studied extensively in FMS patients, perhaps because of the high prevalence of psychological symptoms in this population. While there is considerable variability across studies, rates of depression have been estimated to be as high as 70% (58) and as low as 28.6% (59). It is likely that the actual rate falls somewhere in between [e.g., 34.8% (60); 30% (40)]. Aside from depressive disorders, there is evidence that anxiety disorders (60,61) and posttraumatic stress disorders (62–64) also are prevalent in FMS patients.

Aside from the high incidence of bona fide psychological comorbidities, interest in psychological contributions to FMS has been spurred by the long-standing awareness that FMS patients appraise their symptoms differently than do other rheumatologic patients with similar symptom profiles (40). FMS patients evaluate their symptoms as more severe than do other rheumatologic patients, and they attach greater importance to their symptoms than do other patients. This disordered appraisal process may be centrally mediated: FMS patients demonstrate generally heightened sensitivity to a variety of sensory stimuli (41,65), as well as reduced habituation to such stimuli (66). These and other data suggest that FMS patients are susceptible to augmented pain processing (67). Moreover, augmentation processes appear to be related to levels of psychological distress: higher levels of distress have been shown to mediate activity in brain regions associated with affective aspects of pain processing (68,69).

Given the above, it is not surprising that FMS patients with psychiatric comorbidities also exhibit higher levels of disability and pain-related interference with activity than do patients without such comorbidities (60,62,70). On the other hand, the link between psychiatric disorders and disability in FMS patients is not linear: FMS patients differ not only in their experience of psychiatric disorders, but in the impact that those disorders can have on levels of disability. In fact, several investigative teams have identified clusters of FMS patients who differ in their experience of pain, distress, and disability. One team identified a subset of patients, comprising approximately one-third of the sample, which demonstrated high levels of affective distress, dysfunctional coping responses to pain, and tender point sensitivity (42). Other groups demonstrated moderate or low levels of mood disorders and dysfunction. Another team also identified three distinct subgroups of FMS patients (43). While the subgroups differed somewhat, the most dysfunctional of the groups shared characteristics similar to those described above, including high levels of pain, distress, and disability.

Together, these data suggest that a stress-diathesis model may be a useful heuristic to apply to the FMS disability trajectory. In general, the stress-diathesis model posits that predisposing factors (psychological, genetic, environmental) render some patients vulnerable to negative outcomes following an initiating event (i.e., injury, illness, stress), while other patients exposed to the same event are less vulnerable to such outcomes. [The interested reader is referred to several excellent articles that provide additional detail relative to stress-diathesis models and pain (57,71).] To apply this model to FMS, research to date suggests that a subgroup of patients, characterized by high levels of pain, poor coping, and high levels of distress, may be most likely to exhibit significant functional interference and to develop FMS-related disability. Other groups of FMS patients, characterized either by better coping or lower levels of pain, may be less vulnerable to psychological factors and more vulnerable to other factors (e.g., environmental) relative to the development of disability. If the stress-diathesis model has merit, different approaches to treatment should have differential impact on functional interference and disability across the FMS patient population. The literature bearing on this issue is examined in the next section.

TREATMENT
Given the prevalence and the costs (both personal and societal) of FMS-related disability, treatment strategies that promote functional gains are of great clinical significance. The following sections outline different approaches to the treatment of FMS patients with attention to the impact of treatment on functional interference and disability. The evidence related to single-modality treatments will be examined first, followed by that related to multidisciplinary care.

Single-Modality Treatments
Single-modality approaches to FMS involve a number of treatment types: pharmacotherapy, exercise, education, and cognitive therapy. While complementary and alternative medicine (CAM) also has been used extensively and has exhibited promise (72), the literature regarding the mechanisms that might explain the effectiveness of CAM therapies (acupuncture, biofeedback and relaxation, hypnotherapy, lasers, massage) is limited (73). Hence, that literature is not reviewed here. This section will review literature regarding the pharmacological therapies, then the exercise-oriented therapies, and finally the cognitive therapies, including psychological and/or educational interventions.

Pharmacological Therapies
Antidepressant therapy has constituted the backbone of pharmacological treatment to date, largely because of evidence that it can provide at least modest benefit for FMS symptoms (74,75). Unfortunately, that benefit can diminish with long-term antidepressant administration (76). While opioids and nonsteroidal anti-inflammatory drugs (NSAIDs) would appear to have potential treatment value, data do not support their use except, perhaps, in temporary management of symptoms not primarily related to FMS (77).

Recently, the FDA has approved two drugs for the treatment of fibromyalgia: pregabalin (June 2007) and duloxetine (June 2008), both of which have proved effective in double-blind, placebo-controlled trials. Pregabalin is an α_2-δ ligand with analgesic, anxiolytic, and anticonvulsant activities. It has been shown to be effective in reducing pain, sleep disturbances, and fatigue in FM patients, relative to patients receiving a placebo (35). Improvements also have been documented in patient's perceptions of disability, although the latter effects have not been explicitly investigated with performance-based measures.

Duloxetine is a potent serotonin and norepinephrine reuptake inhibitor that is indicated not only for the treatment of FMS, but also for the treatment of depression, urinary incontinence, and neuropathic pain. In FMS patients with a comorbid major depressive disorder, it has been shown to be effective in reducing the number of tender points and improving the tender point pain threshold as compared to a placebo (34). Given the frequency with which depression is found in FMS patients, as well as the evidence that has shown depression to decrease response to FM treatment (78), the effects with the latter sample are encouraging. The effects of duloxetine on disability in FMS patients are not well studied.

Aside from these FDA-approved therapies, other pharmacological approaches are under study. For example, a short-term study has shown that pyridostigmine, a reversible cholinesterase inhibitor, improves anxiety levels and sleep quality in FMS patients, purportedly through a mechanism involving an increase in vagal tone (79). Similarly, nabilone, a synthetic cannabinoid, has been examined in a four-week trial and has shown preliminary evidence of benefit relative to reported levels of pain severity, anxiety, and self-reported disability (80). While the above studies are only preliminary, they demonstrate the increased interest in pharmacological therapies for FMS patients.

Rehabilitation-Oriented Therapies
Although somewhat dated (it preceded the time of FDA-approved treatments), a three-year longitudinal study found that FM patients perceived non-pharmacological modalities to be more beneficial than pharmacological ones (81). Relative to the issue of FMS disability, the data regarding exercise-oriented therapies are much stronger than the data regarding pharmacological therapies. Indeed, the physical limitations characteristic of FMS patients constitute the rationale for movement-based therapies, addressing such targets as strength deficits of the upper and the lower extremities (82,83), reduced endurance (45), and reduced aerobic capacity (83,84). Aside from the measurable effects of exercise-oriented treatments, a further rationale for involving FMS patients in exercise is evidence that simply occupying patients in some sort of physical activity can distract them from their pain and improve their quality of life (32).

While a variety of exercise approaches have been tried, the best clinical benefits have been found when the fitness program is individually tailored with respect to a patient's baseline physical capacity, severity of symptoms, and pain tolerance (21). Benefits have been found with both aerobic and general conditioning programs that begin with light levels of activity and progress levels of exertion relative to a patient's tolerance. Motivation to continue exercise outside of a supervised environment is a key determinant of long-term benefit. Adjusting an exercise program to the patient's own desires and limitations is fundamental to this goal (85). Such adjustments are of particular importance for patients at high risk of nonadherence, a frequent problem with FMS patients (86). Typically, high-risk patients are those with poor ability to cope with stressors, high levels of upper body pain, practical barriers to exercise (e.g., limited access to exercise facilities), and patients reporting high levels of disability.

Though not all studies of aerobic exercise have found an improvement in patients' aerobic capacity, this may be due to differences between the programs or differences in the patients' baseline physical capacity (85). Nonetheless, the preponderance of studies have demonstrated aerobic benefit from any of a variety of tailored exercise programs, including cycling, dance, whole-body aerobics, walking, and pool exercise (21). Aside from their aerobic benefits, these programs have demonstrated benefits for pain, tender point sensitivity and/or count, self-efficacy, and quality of life (85).

Exercise programs aimed at improving physical capacity also have shown effectiveness in a variety of clinically important dimensions. Progressive strength training—starting from a relatively low load and increasing as function improves—has been shown to increase muscle strength and to reduce symptom severity in FMS patients (85). A recent study utilizing a combined aerobic- and strength-training program demonstrated an improvement in fatigue and fitness for patients with FM (79). As with aerobic exercise programs, there are benefits of performance-based treatments beyond those revealed by physical tests, including increased levels of reported self-efficacy (46).

Cognitive Therapies

Knowledge deficits are widespread among FMS patients: 40% do not have sufficient information to address the question of the possible cause of their symptoms, and 30% see no connection between possible occupational or physical burdens and the course of their disease (87). Such knowledge deficits are thought to contribute to FMS-related dysfunction, secondary to their impact on patients' abilities to manage their health conditions. Consequently, many current FMS treatment programs include an educational component.

Randomized, controlled trials studying the effects of education, however, are relatively few. A meta-analysis of 10 such trials found that they typically offer theoretical information (e.g., current scientific knowledge of FMS, psychosocial influences on pain, the benefits of various treatments), educational discussions (e.g., coping strategies, individualized goal-setting and behavioral strategies), and/or practical discussions (e.g., pain-modifying skills, performing tasks ergonomically). Such classes appear to promote the utilization of pain management strategies and the recognition of the psychosocial impact of FMS, such that they facilitate adjustment to the condition (85).

Psychological therapies also have been employed as FMS treatments, including both operant and cognitive therapies. Operant approaches focus on changing observable pain behaviors through reinforcement of pain-incompatible behavior and extinction of pain behaviors. Cognitive therapies focus on the patient's thinking and problem solving, coping strategies, and relaxation. Cognitive therapies have been shown to influence levels of pain severity, the use of coping strategies, and mood in FMS patients (88), while operant therapies impact functional and behavioral variables as well as pain intensity (89). Both operant and cognitive therapies have been shown to reduce FMS-related disability relative to a more generalized, therapist-guided discussion treatment. As noted earlier, different subsets of patients are likely to respond differentially to cognitive versus operant therapies. In particular, cognitive therapy may be more appropriate for patients who exhibit lower pain behaviors, higher levels of affective distress, and poor coping, while operant therapies may be more beneficial for patients with higher levels of pain behavior and lower levels of distress (90).

Multidisciplinary Treatment

In light of the above studies that document at least modest benefits from various approaches to FMS treatment (pharmacologic, rehabilitative, educational, psychological), it is not surprising that the weight of evidence favors an interdisciplinary approach that combines the therapies (91). The interdisciplinary collaborations can involve only a subset of the above approaches or they can involve all of them. For example, a treatment that combined exercise with education increased exercise tolerance and reduced both postexercise muscle soreness and overuse injuries (92). Similarly, an educational approach that informed patients about the risks and benefits of exercise and how to adjust the exercise to match their own limitations improved adherence to exercise programs (93,94), an important factor in long-term benefit.

For FMS patients who are "both physically and mentally deconditioned" (86), more robust interdisciplinary programs may be needed to improve functional outcomes. While variability in program components and weaknesses in experimental measures and design complicate the interpretation of early studies of multidisciplinary treatment (95), more recent studies suggest that an approach that combines medical, physical, occupational, and psychological therapies may benefit FMS patients (20). An outpatient program that used such components showed significant improvement in levels of pain severity, affective distress, and perceived disability in a patient group characterized by poor coping and high levels of pain and disability (23). Other similarly constituted multidisciplinary treatment studies have demonstrated similar results (92,96). Of equal importance, treatment gains appear to be durable. Relative to standard medical care, a six-week multidisciplinary program involving pharmacology, physical therapy, education, and nutritional guidance yielded significantly improved self-perceived health status, average pain intensity, pain-related disability, depressed affect, and days and hours in pain that persisted at 15-month follow-up (97). In light of these and other studies, current guidelines from the American Pain Society now advocate this approach for the treatment of patients with intransigent FMS (91,98).

DISABILITY DETERMINATION
The previous pages have documented the complex factors that contribute to disability in FMS patients, as well as the value of tailoring treatment to those factors if FMS patients are to improve in their functional capacity. Given the complex picture described above and the frequency with which FMS pain can occasion disability, physicians who treat FMS patients will confront issues related to the medicolegal determination of work disability on a regular basis. In turn, disability determination can be challenging for several reasons. First, FMS is a condition that typically occurs without objective medical evidence to substantiate the severity of reported symptoms (99). Second, psychiatric comorbidities often complicate the clinical picture. Not only do these psychiatric comorbidities raise questions regarding the relative contribution to disability of physical symptoms (e.g., pain, tender points) versus psychiatric symptoms, but they also raise questions about causality (i.e., did the psychiatric problems precede the physical, or vice versa?). Third, the physician who evaluates a patient for disability does so as a last resort, knowing that such a determination comes at a significant price to the patient because disability secondary to pain often presages long-term adjustment problems (17). Hence, a successful disability claim represents a very mixed blessing. Finally, the physician who provides a disability evaluation for an FMS patient does so with the knowledge that the disability determination process can be long and stressful, as such patients often are viewed prejudicially in court settings. Therefore, the claim process can complicate clinical management. Thus, the provider benefits from knowledge about the barriers associated with a disability claim, not only because that knowledge provides guidance regarding factors to be addressed in the evaluation, itself, but because the knowledge can be used to guide the patient through the process, itself. To speak of disability determination as though it is a unitary phenomenon is, of course,

not possible, as there are multiple sources of disability payments, each with its own requirements (15,24). For the purpose of parsimony, this chapter will focus on the disability requirements for Social Security Disability (SSD), although some attention will be paid to interpretations and guidance that have been articulated in cases argued before the federal courts. The following sections will provide a brief history of the criteria for disability determination that have emerged, examine the general attitudes of the courts toward FMS-related disability claims, and discuss the implications of the above for the provider who is conducting a disability determination for an FMS patient.

Historical Issues

The basic judicial test for the determination of disability, the "reasonable man" test, was articulated in findings from the Paul Revere Life Assurance v. Sucharov (1983): "The test of total disability is satisfied when the circumstances are such that a reasonable Man would recognize that he should not engage in certain activity even though he literally is not physically unable to do so." The "reasonable man" reference generally has been interpreted by the courts as imposing an objective standard, often involving the need for objective evidence of a medical condition to support disability claims, irrespective of the severity of the reported symptoms (100). This requirement is reflected in standards adopted by the Social Security Administration which stipulate that disability determination requires the symptoms to be supported by medical signs or findings of a medical condition that could produce those symptoms. Further, they must conform to the following conditions (15): (*i*) disability must prevent gainful employment; (*ii*) work disability must be expected to last at least 12 months; (*iii*) disability must result from a medically determinable physical or mental impairment; and (*iv*) disability must result from anatomical, physiological, or psychological abnormalities that are demonstrable by medically acceptable clinical and laboratory techniques.

Not surprisingly, the need for hard medical evidence to support symptomatic claims has been subject to considerable review and criticism, secondary to the absence of such evidence for many painful conditions, including FM (101,102). Consequently, the adjudication of disability for FMS claims has been subject to revision over the years. While inconsistencies in court findings continue to exist, the trend has gone from strict requirements for medical evidence, often missing in FMS claims, to a standard that attaches greater weight to the contribution of symptoms to disability determination (15, p. 378): ". . . the adjudicator may not discredit the claimant's allegations of the severity of pain solely on the ground that the allegations are unsupported by objective medical evidence." In lieu of strict reliance on medical evidence, a variety of symptom-related factors can be considered that are directly related to FMS pain: (*i*) multiple features of a pain complaint, including its onset, severity, distribution, etc.; (*ii*) factors that exacerbate pain levels; (*iii*) the types and dosages of medications required for pain management; (*iv*) the effectiveness and/or complications from such medications; (*v*) the types of treatments that have been attempted; (*vi*) the level of current functional limitations associated with pain; and (*vii*) the impact of pain on a claimant's usual, daily activities.

The shift in judicial requirements for disability determination is reflected to some degree in changes in the *AMA Guides 5th* related to the assessment of impairment related to pain (25). Where the *Guides* previously have treated pain as largely irrelevant to the assessment of impairment, *AMA Guides 5th* explicitly recognizes that pain and other subjective symptoms can contribute to impairment (*AMA Guides 5th*, p. xx): "An impairment can be manifested objectively, for example, by a fracture, and/or subjectively, through fatigue and pain. Although the *Guides* emphasizes objective assessment, subjective symptoms are included within the diagnostic criteria." Further, it includes a chapter that addresses the assessment of pain-related impairment (103).

While the text of the *AMA Guides 5th* provides latitude for considering pain in the assessment of impairment, there are practical impediments to doing so (102). First, most of the chapters emphasize the application of diagnosis-related estimates that are described as already including such information; this leaves a practitioner uncertain as to whether additional weighting of subjective factors is appropriate. Second, *AMA Guides 5th* instructs practitioners to consider the impact of an injury/illness on activities of daily living (ADLs) as an indicator of impairment. Because this is inconsistent with other definitions of impairment that are organ- and system-based, it is unclear how these perspectives are to be combined. Together, these inconsistencies cloud the assessment of subjective symptoms such as pain and largely obviate the practical benefits of changes in the *AMA Guides 5th* that were intended to address the issue.

In summary, there has been increasing movement toward recognizing subjective symptoms, such as the pain associated with FMS, as contributing to dysfunction and disability. While this movement reduces the need for objective medical evidence to substantiate symptoms, both court opinions and the *AMA Guides 5th* are ambiguous as to how those symptoms are to be considered. This ambiguity has implications for how patients with FMS may be viewed when disability determinations are considered. These implications are addressed in the following section.

Symptom Credibility

As the preceding section indicates, there is ambiguity as to the appropriate weight that FMS-related pain should assume in determination of disability. This ambiguity, combined with the uncertainty associated with such medically unexplained symptoms as FMS, introduces a range of social psychological factors into the determination process (104). This section addresses social psychological factors that may influence how observers view subjective symptoms such as pain, particularly the tendency to underestimate symptom severity. Parallels with the determination of subject credibility in judicial proceedings are also addressed.

Of course, the key question in the determination of pain-related disability is whether an examiner can accurately judge levels of pain and consequent levels of disability that a claimant experiences. While a review of that literature is beyond the scope of this chapter, it is fair to say that the evidence suggests that we cannot. In fact, a range of patient, provider, and situational factors seem to influence judgments. Patient factors that have been shown to occasion the underestimation of pain and influence decisions about pain treatment include young age (105), old age (106), race/ethnicity (56), gender (107), coexisting psychological symptoms (108), the level of reported pain (109,110), and others. Provider factors include level of experience—ironically, more experienced providers discount symptoms to a greater degree than do those with less experience (111)—and area of specialization (112). There also is suggestive evidence that empathy (113) may influence symptom judgments. Finally, situational factors can influence an observer's judgments of pain, including the presence/ absence of litigation (114) and the level of supporting medical evidence (109).

The latter evidence is of particular interest, both because of its relevance to FMS and because of the research that has demonstrated little relationship between objective evidence and levels of pain (115,116). Notwithstanding the latter findings, the absence of supporting medical evidence has been shown consistently to undermine the credibility of symptom reports across a range of observer types: undergraduates (117), medical students (109), and practicing internists (118). Further, practicing medical examiners have shown that they attach substantially greater weight to objective findings than subjective reports (119) when determining pain-related disability. Thus, despite the trend in judicial thinking toward lowering requirements for objective medical evidence and recognizing subjective symptoms as valid contributors to disability, the findings described above suggest that subjective reports of pain continue to be viewed with skepticism.

Data collected on workers' compensation claims over a six-year period (January 1991 to April 1997) in California demonstrate the impediments faced by some classes of disability claimants. The RAND Institute for Social Justice examined impairment ratings, actual earnings loss, and actual benefits received over that time period (120). While the study did not focus on findings relative to pain, results relative to claimants that sustained back injuries are clearly relevant. For claimants with back injuries, especially back injuries with multiple impairments (e.g., impairment of the back and lower extremity, impairment of the back and mental health), the report concluded that examiners were required to rely to a great degree on subjective judgments to determine a claimant's disability. Interestingly, in those cases the impairment ratings provided by claimant physicians exceeded those provided by defense physicians by approximately 90%. Thus, the examiner who must rely on subjective judgments, as is often the case with FMS pain, may be subject to social psychological factors that can influence impairment ratings.

Of course, secondary to concerns about malingering and symptom magnification, there is reason for subjective symptoms to be viewed with some skepticism. In fact, estimates put rates of frank malingering at anywhere from 1.25% to 10% of the patient population (121). That said, it is important to recognize that malingering is a pejorative term that is directly related to a more benign, self-protecting attribute that is common to the population, that is, perception management (122,123): those actions by which people attempt to portray themselves as they want to be seen. In a forensic setting, an extreme form of perception management can involve downright deception; the other end of that extreme, complete transparency, also should be recognized. In truth, most people operate somewhere between those extremes, and how they operate may be determined partly by situational factors.

Relative to the latter point, it is important to recognize that patients with chronic pain often have experienced doubt/skepticism at the hands of the healthcare profession, such that their symptoms may have been attributed to psychological causes (124). In response to these experiences, patients in pain who are sensitive to such matters may present themselves in a manner that emphasizes their physical symptoms and downplays those that are psychological, trying to minimize the likelihood of accusations of psychological causation (125). On a practical basis, it is virtually impossible for providers to discriminate between normal perception management and malingering (126). Indeed, several have argued that examiners who attempt to do so may develop attitudes such that they more often do a disservice to patients with legitimate pain problems than they accurately discern bona fide deception (123,127).

Instead, both these authors and the courts recommend that examiners leave the determination of credibility to the courts (100, p. 32): "The role of the court is to determine plaintiff credibility and whether the impairment results in disability...." A recent study of 194 FMS patients claims that were tried in Canada demonstrated the importance of witness credibility (i.e., agreement of a judge with a plaintiff) in claim settlements (100): highly credible plaintiffs received settlements that were nearly 20 times the size of settlements reached with noncredible plaintiffs. The study also showed the importance of physician/expert testimony in FMS cases: credibility ratings were uniformly higher for experts than for the plaintiffs themselves. Finally, a finding of considerable interest emerged for the relative credibility of treating physicians versus non-treating physicians: treating physicians were significantly more likely to be seen as credible by judges relative to their counterparts.

Clearly, these data suggest that the opinion of a treating physician is valued in the judicial determination of disability. For FMS patients, where objective evidence is often absent and psychiatric comorbidities are common, there are good reasons to value that opinion. First, the treating physician knows whether the patient is a consistent historian and a valid reporter through personal experience. Second, he knows the treatments that a patient has undergone and is undergoing, as well as the patient's general adherence to treatment throughout. Third, he is likely to have a concrete understanding of the patient's everyday activities, the physical demands of the workplace and the home, and the degree to which pain interferes with functioning in each environment. Finally, a treating physician is in a position to appreciate the contribution of psychiatric comorbidities to function. Historically, these comorbidities have been considered to be precipitants of a pain disorder, such that pain often was viewed as psychosomatic. Currently, there is increasing recognition that much psychiatric comorbidity follows pain onset, suggesting a somatopsychic sequence (128). The treating physician is in a unique position to discriminate between the psychosomatic and somatopsychic sequences, a position that the research shows to be recognized by judges.

Disability Evaluation

While the treating physician is well placed to evaluate FMS-related disability, the physician must approach such an evaluation with careful consideration. Such consideration is required for several reasons, one of which involves the unique position that the treating physician faces in the sometimes conflicting roles of treatment provider and disability evaluator. Care also is needed in technical aspects of the evaluation, as some elements of the evaluation are critical if it is to be accorded the validity that it deserves. The following sections review these issues briefly.

Role Considerations

As noted above, the treating physician faces possible conflicts of interest when performing a disability evaluation for a patient/claimant. This is less an issue for patients for whom a disability application is truly the last resort: they have partnered in a range of failed treatments and attempted vainly to maintain a productive functional status. In those cases, the treating physician can provide a straightforward evaluation that will honestly advocate disability. For other patients, such as those who have pursued treatment half-heartedly and/or who demonstrate dysfunctional coping strategies despite intervention, the potential for conflicts of interest is more problematic. Because the treating physician no longer can address the self-defeating patterns with the hope of clinical benefit, the disability application is more frustrating here than in the former case.

In the latter case, should the patient insist on pursuing a disability claim despite countervailing arguments, the physician has only two choices. In extreme cases, he or she can refuse to perform the disability evaluation and/or inform the patient that the evaluation will not further the disability claim. Even here, however, the physician may receive a court request for records and an opinion regarding the patient's pain-related function. Alternatively, the physician can adopt a neutral attitude and provide a descriptive clinical picture. This approach acknowledges the reality of a disability claim: the courts decide the severity of the disability and the credibility of the claim.

Technical Considerations

Of course, defining disability represents a dilemma with FMS patients, especially as disability status cannot be affixed by reference to objective indices of impairment. Criteria applicable to FM have been proposed that are key to the concept of work disability (15): (*i*) consistent work attendance, (*ii*) acceptable work quality, and (*iii*) adequate response to supervision and/or criticism. When patients demonstrate discontinuous work attendance (e.g., five or more missed days/month) and/or work of poor quality irrespective of supervision, they may qualify for determination of work disability secondary to FMS.

An obvious element of an FMS disability evaluation involves a description of the patient's current symptom status. This should include assessment of the severity of both physical (pain severity, tender points, pain distribution, fatigue) and psychological (depression, anxiety) symptoms. Relative to pain, it is useful to provide information regarding levels of worst, least, and usual pain, using instruments with established measurement properties. The duration of symptom exacerbations also should be noted, as a patient who experiences brief, intermittent exacerbations is qualitatively different than one who experiences prolonged pain exacerbations. Further, the evaluation should document the time course of the symptoms, including the circumstances of pain onset. While the need for such information is obvious in circumstances where pain onset follows trauma, it also is important when onset is more insidious. Of course, treatment history also should be included, citing not only the therapies that have been tried, but also the level of treatment adherence that the patient has demonstrated.

Of course, it is important to recognize that disability systems are grounded in objective medical evidence, typically defined as abnormalities detectable on X ray, MRI, EMG, etc. Therefore, it is crucial for the disability evaluation to include

TABLE 1 Semiobjective Findings on Physical Examination

1. Abnormal posture (e.g., list)
2. Abnormal gait
3. Muscle spasm
4. Hypersensitivity (tender points)
5. Reduced range of motion
6. Abnormal straight leg raising
7. Reduced sensory function in extremities
8. Reduced extremity strength

documentation of the signs and symptoms that establish an FMS diagnosis, using the 1990 ACR criteria. This medical documentation is essential, as simple assertions that symptoms are consistent with a diagnosis of FM may be inadequate, especially in the (many) instances where FMS patients are seen by specialists who are likely to assert other diagnoses. Of course, hard abnormal objective findings often are lacking in FMS. Even when present, they may fail to capture the extent of functional interference associated with the disorder. Robinson (24) recommends that practitioners, instead, consider describing a range of "semiobjective findings" that may be used as proxies for the "harder" objective findings (Table 1).

FMS-related functional interference also must be established, typically by reference to the impact of FMS on everyday work and home roles. Indeed, the *AMA Guides 5th* suggest that interference with ADL functions can be used as an indicator of pain-related impairment. Unfortunately, the *Guides* fail to provide criteria by which to evaluate ADL performance. Thus, the examiner may be faced with estimating the degree to which work is impacted, a determination that is made more straightforward if the examiner knows the number of days in an average month that pain, fatigue, and psychological distress interfere with work activity, as well as the efforts at work accommodation that have been made. Such information also can guide decisions as to whether the patient is partially or totally disabled.

CONCLUDING REMARKS

Clearly, recent years have seen substantial progress in the management of disability associated with FMS. Research, both basic and applied, has given us a better understanding of the syndrome and has directed attention from peripheral to central mechanisms. This research also has clarified why peripherally acting agents (e.g., NSAIDs) have not proved effective, while centrally acting agents (e.g., antidepressants) have done so. Similarly, lines of research have identified clusters of FMS patients who have clinically different profiles; these profiles appear useful in tailoring interventions so that they provide optimal impact. Clearly, we can expect that further advances in our understanding of FMS mechanisms will continue to translate into improved clinical applications.

While progress has been made in understanding FMS mechanisms, the management of disability in this patient group continues to be challenging. The management of the complex symptoms that can characterize the syndrome can overwhelm the resources of a single practitioner. At the same time, access to interdisciplinary treatment, the preferred option for patients with intransigent symptoms (91), continues to decrease as the fiscal viability of many such centers has been eroded by changes in insurance reimbursement (129). The net effect is that, despite the abundant progress, too many patients continue along a clinical trajectory that leads to disability.

What steps are available to the individual practitioner who might modify the course of that trajectory? Probably the most important step involves guarding against the disbelief that has been shown to attend the treatment of patients with medically unexplained symptoms (130). When disbelief governs practice, one of two unproductive options is usually obtained: (*i*) unnecessary diagnostic tests are ordered in an (unsuccessful) effort to find objective validation of symptoms, or (*ii*) standard care is rendered as a default option with its predictably negative implications for the clinical course. An alternative (albeit more laborious) approach involves thorough assessment of the medical, functional, and psychosocial problems that these patients can present and then partnering with patients in an appropriately tailored, yet functionally oriented program of care (90).

While the data suggest that either physical conditioning or aerobic exercise should constitute an element of their treatment, other needs are likely to differ. For some, pain will represent the greatest threat to loss of function; others will face threats from fatigue or psychiatric comorbidities. Those practitioners fortunate enough to have access to primary care psychological services may have sufficient resources to manage the patients in their offices. Those practitioners with access to interdisciplinary pain services have a ready referral for coordinated care. Those who do not must identify both rehabilitation and mental health providers in the surrounding community, preferably with expertise in the treatment of FMS. Failure to address the various comorbidities that can attend FMS is likely to undermine functional progress that otherwise would occur.

Of course, the above recommendations are predicated on the belief that interdisciplinary care is not only the optimal approach to the treatment of FMS patients, but also an approach that can yield long-term functional benefits. Truthfully, the data that support this assumption remain somewhat weak, as they are based on modest effects in small samples generally measured over limited time periods (95). Recent advances aimed at tailoring treatment show more robust effects, but long-term data still are needed to support the cost-benefit value of these labor-intensive programs (20,97).

Aside from the need for data bearing on the long-term durability of interdisciplinary treatment, guidance is needed in the disability determination arena, particularly the correspondence among impairment ratings, court-rendered disability ratings, and the long-term functional status of FMS claimants that filed disability claims. Suggestive data derived from studies of occupational low back pain show little relationship between indicators of impairment, disability ratings, and long-term adjustment (131). Similar studies with FMS patients could be instructive for providers who conduct disability evaluations, particularly when they are required to provide objective evidence (and/or semiobjective evidence) that may bear little relationship to the matter being heard (i.e., a claimant's long-term functional status). Present-day requirements, derived from an impairment-based system with known flaws, may actually interfere with reasonable decision-making.

In summary, advances in our clinical understanding of FMS offer patients and providers with more hope for symptom control and functional gains than was possible even a few years ago. Paradigms for treatment tailored to the individual needs of a patient appear promising. The implementation of those paradigms, however, requires not only an informed physician, but access to a variety of disciplines that can promote increased function and improved coping. Unfortunately, access to and coordination of these disciplines can be problematic, and access to interdisciplinary facilities even more so as their numbers diminish. Until a more rational approach can be adopted on a national level, disability management in FMS, always challenging, will remain more challenging than it has to be.

ACKNOWLEDGMENT

The development of this manuscript was supported in part by grant # R01 HS 14007 from the Agency for Healthcare Research and Quality.

REFERENCES

1. White KP, Speechley M, Harth M, et al. The London Fibromyalgia Epidemiology Study: the prevalence of fibromyalgia syndrome in London, Ontario. J Rheumatol 1999; 26:1570–1576.
2. Wolfe F, Ross K, Anderson J, et al. The prevalence and characteristics of fibromyalgia in the general population. Arthritis Rheum 1995; 38:19–28.
3. Wolfe F, Smythe HA, Yunus MB, et al. The American College of Rheumatology 1990 criteria for the classification of fibromyalgia: report of the multicenter criteria committee. Arthritis Rheum 1990; 33:160–172.
4. Lawrence RC, Felson DT, Helmick CG, et al. Estimates of the prevalence of arthritis and other rheumatic conditions in the United States: part II. Arthritis Rheum 2008; 58:26–35.
5. White KP, Carette S, Harth M, et al. Trauma and fibromyalgia: is there an association and what does it mean? Semin Arthritis Rheum 2000; 29:200–216.
6. Goldenberg DL. Fibromyalgia syndrome a decade later: what have we learned? Arch Intern Med 1999; 159:777–785.
7. Kosek E, Edholm J, Hansson P. Increased pressure pain sensibility in fibromyalgia patients is located deep in the skin but not restricted to muscle tissue. Pain 1995; 63:335–339.
8. Pillemer SR, Bradley LA, Crofford LJ, et al. Conference summary: the neuroscience and endocrinology of fibromyalgia. Arthritis Rheum 1997; 40:1928–1939.
9. Katz RS, Wolfe F, Michaud K. Fibromyalgia diagnosis: a comparison of clinical, survey, and American College of Rheumatology criteria. Arthritis Rheum 2006; 54(1):69–176.
10. Wolfe F. The relation between tender points and fibromyalgia symptom variables: evidence that fibromyalgia is not a discrete disorder in the clinic. Ann Rheum Dis 1997; 56:268–271.
11. Ahles TA, Khan SA, Yunus MB, et al. Psychiatric status of patients with primary fibromyalgia, patients with rheumatoid arthritis, and subjects without pain: a blind comparison of DSM-III diagnosis. Am J Psychiatry 1991; 148:1721–1726.
12. Hudson JI, Goldenberg DL, Pope HG Jr., et al. Comorbidity of fibromyalgia with medical and psychiatric disorders. Am J Med 1992; 92:363–367.
13. Sayar K, Gulec H, Topbas M, et al. Affective distress and fibromyalgia. Swiss Med Wkly 2004; 134:248–253.
14. Panton LB, Kingsley JD, Toole T, et al. A comparison of physical functional performance and strength in women with fibromyalgia, age- and weight-matched controls, and older women who are healthy. Phys Ther 2006; 86:1479–1488.
15. Wolfe F, Potter J. Fibromyalgia and work disability: is fibromyalgia a disabling disorder? Rheum Dis Clin North Am 1996; 22:370–391.
16. Wolfe F, Anderson J, Harkness D, et al. Work and disability status of persons with fibromyalgia. J Rheumatol 1997; 24(6):1171–1178.

17. Von Korff M, Deyo RA, Cherkin D, et al. Back pain in primary care. Outcomes at 1 year. Spine 1993; 18:855–862.
18. Ledingham J, Doherty S, Doherty M. Primary fibromyalgia syndrome—an outcome study. Br J Rheumatol 1993; 32:139–142.
19. Wolfe F, Anderson J, Harkness D, et al. Health status and disease severity in fibromyalgia: results of a six-center longitudinal study. Arthritis Rheum 1997; 40(9):1571–1579.
20. Adams N, Sim J. Rehabilitation approaches in fibromyalgia. Disabil Rehabil 2005; 27:711–723.
21. Mannerkorpi K. Exercise in fibromyalgia. Curr Opin Rheumatol 2005; 17:190–194.
22. Nielson WR, Jensen MP. Relationship between changes in coping and treatment outcome in patients with fibromyalgia syndrome. Pain 2004; 109:233–241.
23. Turk DC, Okifuji A, Sinclair JD, et al. Differential responses by psychosocial subgroups of fibromyalgia syndrome patients to an interdisciplinary treatment. Arthritis Care Res 1998; 11:397–404.
24. Robinson JP. Disability evaluation in painful conditions. In: Turk DC, Melzack R, eds. Handbook of Pain Assessment. 2nd ed. New York: The Guilford Press, 2001:248–272.
25. Cocchiarella L, Andersson GBJ, eds. Guides to the Evaluation of Permanent Impairment. 5th ed. Chicago, IL: AMA Press, 2001.
26. Wolfe F, Anderson J, Harkness D, et al. A prospective, longitudinal, multicenter study of service utilization and costs in fibromyalgia. Arthritis Rheum, 1997; 40: 1560–1570.
27. Cathey MA, Wofe F, Roberts FK, et al. Demographics, work disability, service utilization and treatment characteristics of 620 fibromyalgia patients in rheumatologic practice. Arthritis Rheum 1990; 33 (suppl 9):S10 (abstr).
28. Al-Allaf AW. Work disability and health system utilization in patients with fibromyalgia syndrome. J Clin Rheum 2007; 13:199–201.
29. Brunsgaard D, Evensen AR, Bjerkedal T. Fibromyalgia—a new cause for disability pension. Scand J Soc Med 1993; 21:116–119.
30. McCain GA, Cameron R, Kennedy JC. The problem of long term disability payments and litigation in primary fibromyalgia: the Canadian perspective. J Rheumatol 1989; 16(suppl 19):147–176.
31. Bengtsson A, Backman E, Lindblom B, et al. Long-term follow-up of fibromyalgia patients: clinical symptoms, muscular function, laboratory tests—an eight year comparison study. J Musculoskel Pain 1994; 2:67–80.
32. Wigers SH. Fibromyalgia outcome: the predictive values of symptom duration, physical activity, disability pension, and critical life events—a 4.5 year prospective study. J Psychosom Res 1996; 41:235–243.
33. White KP, Nielson WR, Harth M, et al. Does the label "fibromyalgia" alter health status, function, and health service utilization? A prospective, within-group comparison in a community cohort of adults with chronic widespread pain. Arthritis Rheum 2002; 47:260–265.
34. Arnold LM, Lu Y, Crofford LJ, et al. A double-blind, multicenter trial comparing duloxetine with placebo in the treatment of fibromyalgia with or without major depressive disorder. Arthritis Rheum 2004; 50(9):2974–2984.
35. Crofford LJ, Rowbotham MC, Mease PJ, et al. Pregabalin for the treatment of fibromyalgia syndrome: results of a randomized, double-blind, placebo-controlled trial. Arthritis Rheum 2005; 52(4):1264–1273.
36. Vollestad NK, Mengshoel AN. Relationships between neuromuscular functioning, disability and pain in fibromyalgia. Disabil Rehabil 2005; 27:667–673.
37. Hadler NM. If you have to prove you are ill, you can't get well: the object lesson of fibromyalgia. Spine 1996; 21:2397–2400.
38. Hadler NM. Fibromyalgia: La maladie est moret. Vive la malade! J Rheumatol 1997; 24:1250–1252.
39. Robbins JM, Kirmayer LJ, Kapusta MA. Illness, worry and disability in fibromyalgia syndrome. Intl J Psych Med 1990; 20:49–63.

40. Wolfe F, Hawley DJ. Evidence of disordered symptom appraisal in fibromyalgia: increased rates of reported comorbidity and comorbidity severity. Clin Exp Rheumatol 1999; 17:297–303.
41. Geisser ME, Glass JM, Rajcevska LD, et al. A psychophysical study of auditory and pressure sensitivity in patients with fibromyalgia and healthy controls. J Pain 2008; 9:417–422.
42. Giesecke T, Williams DA, Harris RE, et al. Subgrouping of fibromyalgia patients on the basis of pressure-pain thresholds and psychological factors. Arthritis Rheum 2003; 48:2916–2922.
43. Turk DC, Okifuji A, Sinclair JD, et al. Pain, disability and physical functioning in subgroups of patients with fibromyalgia. J Rheumatol 1996; 23:1255–1262.
44. De Gier M, Peters ML, Vlaeyen JWS. Fear of pain, physical performance and attentional processes in patients with fibromyalgia. Pain 2003; 104:121–130.
45. Kop WJ, Lyden A, Berlin AA, et al. Ambulatory monitoring of physical activity and symptoms in fibromyalgia and chronic fatigue syndrome. Arthritis Rheum 2005; 52:296–303.
46. Mannerkorpi K, Svantesson U, Broberg C. Relationships between performance-based tests and patients' ratings of activity limitations, self-efficacy, and pain in fibromyalgia. Arch Phys Med Rehabil 2006; 87:259–264.
47. Gheldof ELM, Vinck J, Vlaeyen JWS, et al. The differential role of pain, work characteristics and pain-related fear in explaining back pain and sick leave in occupational settings. Pain 2005; 113:71–81.
48. Liedberg GM, Henriksson CM. Factors of importance for work disability in women with fibromyalgia: an interview study. Arthritis Rheum 2002; 47:266–274.
49. Henriksson CM, Liedberg GM, Gerdle B. Women with fibromyalgia: work and rehabilitation. Disabil Rehabil 2005; 27:685–695.
50. Wolfe F, Hawley DJ, Wilson K. The prevalence and meaning of fatigue in rheumatic disease. J Rheumatol 1996; 23:1407–1417.
51. Nicassio PM, Moxham EG, Schuman CE, et al. The contribution of pain, reported sleep quality, and depressive symptoms to fatigue in fibromyalgia. Pain 2002; 100:271–279.
52. Teasell RW, Merskey H. Chronic pain disability in the work place. Am Pain Forum 1997; 6:228–238.
53. Gheldof ELM, Vinck J, Vlaeyen JWS, et al. The differential role of pain, work characteristics and pain-related fear in explaining back pain and sick leave in occupational settings. Pain 2005; 113:71–81.
54. Henriksson C, Liedberg G. Factors of importance for work disability in women with fibromyalgia. J Rheumatol 2000; 27:171–176.
55. Teasell RW, Bombardier C. Employment-related factors in chronic pain and chronic pain disability. Clin J Pain 2001; 17:S39–S45.
56. Green CR, Anderson KO, Baker TA, et al. The unequal burden of pain: confronting racial and ethnic disparities in pain. Pain Med 2003; 4:277–294.
57. Turk DC. A diathesis-stress model of chronic pain and disability following traumatic injury. Pain Res Manage 2002; 7:9–19.
58. Epstein SA, Kay G, Claux D, et al. Psychiatric disorders in patients with fibromyalgia. Psychosomatics 1999; 40:57–63.
59. Ahles TA, Yunus MB, Masi AT. Is chronic pain a variant of depressive disease? The case of primary fibromyalgia syndrome. Pain 1987; 29:105–111.
60. Thieme K, Turk DC, Flor H. Comorbid depression and anxiety in fibromyalgia syndrome: relationship to somatic and psychosocial variables. Psychosom Med 2004; 66:837–844.
61. Sayar K, Gulec H, Topbas M, et al. Affective distress and fibromyalgia. Swiss Med Wkly 2004; 134:248–253.
62. Sherman JJ, Turk DC, Okifuji A. Prevalence and impact of posttraumatic stress disorder-like symptoms on patients with fibromyalgia syndrome. Clin J Pain 2000; 16:127–134.

63. Walker EA, Keegan D, Gardner G, et al. Psychosocial factors in fibromyalgia compared with rheumatoid arthritis: I. Psychiatric diagnoses and functional disability. Psychosom Med 1997; 59:565–571.
64. Walker EA, Keegan D, Gardner G, et al. Psychosocial factors in fibromyalgia compared with rheumatoid arthritis: II. Sexual, physical, and emotional abuse and neglect. Psychosom Med 1997; 59:572–577.
65. McDermid AJ, Rollman GB, McCain GA. Generalized hypervigilance in fibromyalgia: evidence of perceptual amplification. Pain 1996; 66:133–144.
66. Montoya P, Sitges C, Garcia-Herrera M, et al. Reduced brain habituation to somatosensory stimulation in patients with fibromyalgia. Arthritis Rheum 2006; 54:1995–2003.
67. Gracely RH, Petzke F, Wolf JM, et al. Functional magnetic resonance imaging evidence of augmented pain processing in fibromyalgia. Arthritis Rheum 2002; 46:1333–1343.
68. Giesecke T, Gracely RH, Williams DA, et al. The relationship between depression, clinical pain, and experimental pain in a chronic pain cohort. Arthritis Rheum 2005; 52:1577–1584.
69. Petzke F, Gracely RH, Park KM, et al. What do tender points measure? Influence of distress on 4 measures of tenderness. J Rheumatol 2003; 30:567–574.
70. Verbunt JA, Pernot DH, Smeets RJ. Disability and quality of life in patients with fibromyalgia. Health Qual Life Outcomes 2008; 6:8; (doi:10.1186/1477-7525-6-8).
71. Chapman CR, Tuckett RP, Song CW. Pain and stress in a systems perspective: reciprocal neural, endocrine, and immune interactions. J Pain 2008; 9:122–145.
72. Eisenberg DM, Davis RB, Ettner SL, et al. Trends in alternative medicine use in the United States, 1990–1997. JAMA 1998; 280(18):1569–1575.
73. Harris RE, Clauw DJ. The use of complementary medical therapies in the management of myofascial pain disorders. Curr Pain Headache Rep 2002; 6:370–374.
74. Arnold LM, Keck PE Jr., Welge JA. Antidepressant treatment of fibromyalgia: a meta-analysis and review. Psychosomatics 2000; 41:104–113.
75. Leventhal LJ. Management of fibromyalgia. Ann Intern Med 1999; 131(11):850–858.
76. Carette S, Bell MJ, Reynolds WJ, et al. Comparison of amitriptyline, cyclobenzaprine, and placebo in the treatment of fibromyalgia: a randomized, double-blind clinical trial. Arthritis Rheum 1994; 37:32–40.
77. Goldenberg DL, Burckhardt C, Crofford L. Management of fibromyalgia syndrome. JAMA 2004; 292:2388–2395.
78. Finset A, Wigers SH, Götestam KG. Depressed mood impedes pain treatment response in patients with fibromyalgia. J Rheumatol 2004; 31(5):976–980.
79. Jones KD, Burckhardt CS, Deodhar AA, et al. A six-month randomized controlled trial of exercise and pyridostigmine in the treatment of fibromyalgia. Arthritis Rheum 2008; 58(2):612–622.
80. Skrabek RQ, Galimova L, Ethans K, et al. Nabilone for the treatment of pain in fibromyalgia. J Pain 2008; 9:164–173.
81. Pöyhiä R, Da Costa D, Fitzcharles M. Pain and pain relief in fibromyalgia patients followed for three years. Arthritis Rheum 2001; 45(4):355–361.
82. Mannerkorpi K, Burckhardt CS, Bjelle A. Physical performance characteristics of women with fibromyalgia. Arthritis Care Res 1994; 7:123–129.
83. Mengshoel AM, Forre O, Komnaes HB. Muscle strength and aerobic capacity in primary fibromyalgia. Clin Exp Rheumatol 1990; 8:475–479.
84. Nielens H, Boisset V, Masquerlier E. Fitness and perceived exertion in patients with fibromyalgia syndrome. Clin J Pain 2000; 16(3):209–213.
85. Mannerkorpi K, Henrikson C. Non-pharmological treatment of chronic widespread musculoskeletal pain. Best Pract Res Clin Rheumatol 2007; 21(3):513–534.
86. Dobkin PL, Abrahamowicz M, Fitzcharles M, et al. Maintenance of exercise in women with fibromyalgia. Arthritis Care Res 2005; 53(5):724–731.
87. Nöller V, Sprott H. Prospective epidemiological observations on the course of disease in fibromyalgia patients. J Negat Results Biomed 2003; 2:4. Available at: http://www.jnrbm.com/content/2/1/4

88. Thieme K, Flor H, Turk DC. Psychological pain treatment in fibromyalgia syndrome: efficacy of operant behavioural and cognitive behavioural treatments. Arthritis Res Ther 2006; 8:R121. Available at: http://arthritis-research.com/content/8/4/r121
89. Thieme K, Gromnica-Ihle E, Flor H. Operant behavioral treatment of fibromyalgia: a controlled study. Arthritis Care Res 2003; 49(3):314–320.
90. Thieme K, Turk DC, Flor H. Responder criteria for operant and cognitive-behavioral treatment of fibromyalgia syndrome. Arthritis Care Res 2007; 57(5):830–836.
91. Burckhardt C, Goldenberg DL, Crofford L. Guideline for the management of fibromyalgia syndrome pain in adults and children. APS Clinical Practice Guidelines Series, No. 4. Chicago, IL: American Pain Society, 2005.
92. Wennemer HK, Borg-Stein J, Gomba L, et al. Functionally oriented rehabilitation program for patients with fibromyalgia: preliminary results. Am J Phys Med Rehabil 2006; 85(8):659–666.
93. Iversen MD, Eaton HM, Daltroy LH. How rheumatologists and patients with rheumatoid arthritis discuss exercise and the influence of discussions on exercise prescriptions. Arthritis Rheum 2004; 51(1):63–72.
94. Mannerkorpi K, Ahlmen M, Ekdahl C. Six and 24-month follow up of pool exercise and education for patients with fibromyalgia. Scand J Rheumatol 2002; 31:306–310.
95. Sim J, Adams N. Systematic review of randomized controlled trials of non-pharmacological interventions for fibromyalgia. Clin J Pain 2002; 18:324–336.
96. Angst F, Brioshci R, Main CJ, et al. Interdisciplinary rehabilitation in fibromyalgia and chronic back pain: a prospective outcome study. J Pain 2006; 7:807–815.
97. Lemstra M, Olszynski WP. The effectiveness of multidisciplinary rehabilitation in the treatment of fibromyalgia; a randomized controlled trial. Clin J Pain 2005; 21(2):166–174.
98. Turk DC, Vierck CJ, Scarbrough E, et al. Fibromyalgia: combining pharmacological and nonpharmacological approaches to treating the person, not just the pain. J Pain 2008; 9:99–104.
99. Aaron LA, Buchwald D. A review of the evidence for overlap among unexplained clinical conditions. Ann Intern Med 2001; 134:868–881.
100. Le Page JA, Iverson GL, Collins P. The impact of judges' perceptions of credibility in fibromyalgia claims. Int J Law Psychiat 2008; 31:30–40.
101. Osterweis M, Kleinman A, Mechanic D, eds. Pain and Disability. Washington, D.C.: National Academy Press, 1987.
102. Robinson JP, Turk DC, Loeser JD. Pain, impairment, and disability in the AMA Guides. J Law Med Ethics 2004; 32:315–326.
103. Turk DC, Robinson JP, Loeser JD, et al. Pain. In: Cocchiarella L, Andersson GBJ, eds. Guides to the Evaluation of Permanent Impairment. 5th ed. Chicago, Illinois: AMA Press, 2001:565–591.
104. Tait RC, Chibnall JT, Kalauokalani D. Provider judgments of patients in pain: seeking symptom certainty. Pain Med 2009: 11–34.
105. Hamers JPH, Abu-Saad HH, van den Hout MA, et al. The influence of children's vocal expressions, age, medical diagnosis and information obtained from parents on nurses' pain assessments and decisions regarding interventions. Pain 1996; 65:53–61.
106. Teno JM, Weitzen S, Wetle T, et al. Persistent pain in nursing home residents. JAMA 2001; 285:2081.
107. McDonald DD, Bridge RG. Gender stereotyping and nursing care. Res Nurs Health 1991; 143:373–378.
108. Elander J, Marczewska M, Amos R, et al. Factors affecting hospital staff judgments about sickle cell disease. J Behav Med 2006; 29:203–214.
109. Chibnall JT, Tait RC, Ross L. The effects of medical evidence and pain intensity on medical student judgments of chronic pain patients. J Behav Med 1997; 20:257–271.
110. Grossman SA, Sheidler VR, Swedeen K, et al. Correlation of patient and caregiver ratings of cancer pain. J Pain Symptom Manage 1991; 6:53–57.
111. Marquie L, Raufaste E, Lauque D, et al. Pain rating by patients and physicians: evidence of systematic pain miscalibration. Pain 2003; 102:289–296.

112. Chibnall JT, Tait RC, Merys S. Disability management of low back injuries by employer-retained physicians: ratings and costs. Am J Ind Med 2000; 38:529–538.
113. Tait RC, Chibnall JT, Luebbert A, et al. Effect of treatment success and empathy on surgeon attributions for back surgery outcomes. J Behav Med 2005; 28:301–312.
114. Tait RC, Chibnall JT. Observer perceptions of chronic low back pain. J Appl Soc Psychol 1994; 24:415–431.
115. Jensen CJ, Brant-Zawaszki MN, Obuchowski N, et al. Magnetic resonance imaging of the lumbar spine in people without back pain. N Engl J Med 1994; 331:69–73.
116. Michel A, Kohlmann T, Raspe H. The association between clinical findings on physical examination and self-reported severity in back pain. Spine 1997; 22:296–304.
117. Tait RC, Chibnall JT. Observer perceptions of chronic low back pain. J Appl Soc Psychol 1994; 24:415–431.
118. Tait RC, Chibnall JT. Physician judgments of patients with intractable low back pain. Soc Sci Med 1997; 45:1199–1205.
119. Carey TS, Hadler NM, Gillings D, et al. Medical disability assessment of the back pain patient for the Social Security Administration: the weighting of presenting clinical features. J Clin Epidemiol 1988; 41:691–697.
120. Reville RT, Seabury SA, Neuhauser FW, et al. An Evaluation of California's Permanent Disability Rating System. Santa Monica, CA: RAND Corporation, MG-258, 2005.
121. Fishbain DA, Cutler R, Rosomoff HL, et al. Chronic pain disability exaggeration/malingering and submaximal effort research. Clin J Pain 1999; 15:244–274.
122. Goffman E. The Presentation of Self in Everyday Life. Garden City, NY: Doubleday, 1959.
123. Mendelson G, Mendelson D. Malingering pain in the medicolegal context. Clin J Pain 2004; 20:423–432.
124. Marbach JJ, Lennon MC, Link BG, et al. Losing face: sources of stigma perceived by chronic facial pain patients. J Behav Med 1990; 13:583–604.
125. Deshields TL, Tait RC, Gfeller JD, et al. The relationship between social desirability and self-report in chronic pain patients. Clin J Pain 1995; 11:189–193.
126. Hill ML, Craig KD. Detecting deception in pain expressions: the structure of genuine and deceptive facial displays. Pain 2002; 98:135–144.
127. Craig KD, Badali MA. Introduction to the special series on pain deception and malingering. Clin J Pain 2004; 20:377–382.
128. Dersh J, Mayer T, Theodore BR, et al. Do psychiatric disorders first appear preinjury or postinjury in chronic disabling occupational spinal disorders? Spine 2007; 32:1045–1051.
129. Schatman ME. The demise of the multidisciplinary chronic pain management clinic: bioethical perspectives on providing optimal treatment when ethical principles collide. In: Schatman ME, ed. Ethical Issues in Chronic Pain Management. New York: Informa Healthcare, 2007.
130. Epstein RM, Shields CG, Meldrum SC, et al. Physicians' responses to patients' medically unexplained symptoms. Psychosom Med 2006; 68:269–276.
131. Tait RC, Chibnall JT, Andresen EA, et al. Disability determination: validity with occupational low back pain. J Pain 2006; 7:951–957.

7 Exercise as an Intervention for Individuals with Fibromyalgia

S. E. Gowans
Allied Health, University Health Network; Department of Physical Therapy, University of Toronto, Toronto, Ontario, Canada

A. deHueck
Physiotherapy Department, Joseph Brant Memorial Hospital, Burlington, Ontario, Canada

INTRODUCTION

The first randomized, controlled study on the merits of exercise for individuals with fibromyalgia (FM) was published in the late 1980s (1). This seminal study, which compared the merits of 20 weeks of aerobic exercise with 20 weeks of stretching, indicated that aerobic exercise could produce greater improvements in physical fitness, tender point pain, and patient/physician global assessment ratings than stretching alone. Since then many studies have examined the benefits of exercise for individuals with FM (for a comprehensive listing of studies prior to Jan 2006 see Ref. 2) and several meta-analyses have been conducted (for the most recent meta-analysis see Ref. 3).

BENEFITS OF DIFFERENT TYPES OF EXERCISE
Aerobic Exercise

Aerobic exercise has received the most scrutiny, in terms of both the number of studies and the number of meta-analyses that have been conducted.

The most recent meta-analysis on exercise and FM concluded that moderately intense aerobic exercise for 6 to 23 weeks can improve physical function and global well-being (3). The same meta-analysis implied that moderately intense aerobic exercise *may* also improve pain and tender points since large improvements in pain and small improvements in tender points were seen, but neither of these improvements was statistically significant (3).

Significant improvements in physical function with aerobic exercise are important since individuals with FM are often physically unfit (4). Increasing physical function may stop the downward spiral whereby pain leads to decreased physical activity, which causes muscle weakness, and then individuals experience increased pain with the same or lower levels of physical activity, and do less, etc. Further, although improvements in pain were not significant in the meta-analysis, the fact that aerobic exercise did not *increase* pain is noteworthy because individuals with FM fear that exercise will exacerbate their pain.

Do these improvements last? Typically, subjects have been monitored for one year or less following the end of supervised aerobic exercise classes, although one study followed patients for 4.5 years (5). Studies indicate that immediate gains, particularly in physical function, can be maintained, but ongoing exercise may be required for ongoing benefit, since follow-up studies indicate a positive relationship between ongoing exercise adherence and the maintenance of exercise-induced changes (5–7). The fact that ongoing exercise is required for ongoing benefit is not surprising, especially if the improvements are in physical function, since exercise-induced gains in cardiovascular fitness are known to be lost once exercise has stopped for four weeks (8).

Strengthening

Strengthening, especially strengthening in isolation, has received much less scrutiny than aerobic exercise. To date, four randomized control trials have been conducted on the effects of strengthening alone versus no exercise or stretching for individuals with FM (9–12). Three of these studies evaluated intensive strengthening programs on specialized equipment, where the resistance for each exercise was individually determined. Participants in the fourth study did arm and leg exercises as a group, against resistance from gravity or elastic tubing or hand-held weights (10). This fourth study is similar to community-based strengthening programs that are run in a group format, without specialized strengthening equipment. Only the three intensive strengthening programs produced significant gains in muscle strength in exercising compared to that in control subjects. None of the four strengthening programs increased pain.

The recent meta-analysis, with data from two of the four strengthening studies, concluded that there was some/limited evidence that strengthening could improve pain, global well-being, tender points, and depression (3). Medium-sized improvements in physical function were noted in the same meta-analysis, but these improvements, with a limited data set, were not significant (3).

Whether the benefits of strengthening persist is unknown, since follow-up data has not been gathered.

Stretching

Stretching has not been studied as an exercise intervention but has been used as a control condition for several exercise trials (1,10). Although stretching produced some short-term improvements in study outcomes, stretching produced fewer improvements than aerobic exercise or strengthening in the same trials. Improvements following stretching suggest that either stretching itself is therapeutic or that study outcomes were improved following stretching due to other factor(s) (e.g., social support from the exercise classes, passage of time, familiarity with tests, etc.).

Qigong and Tai Chi

Qigong and Tai Chi are forms of low-intensity exercise that have received limited scrutiny: in terms of both the numbers of studies conducted and/or the methodological strength of the studies themselves.

Three randomized controlled trials have compared Qigong (a Chinese healthcare system that combines specific postures with breathing techniques and focused intention) with/without mindful meditation to usual care (13,14) or an educational support group (15). The results of these three Qigong studies are mixed. The first study that compared three months of Qigong to usual care found no improvements in functional measures or a disease-specific measure (Fibromyalgia Impact Questionnaire), although the Qigong group had better movement quality on an objective scale. The second study that compared eight weeks of Qigong plus mindful meditation to an educational support group found that both interventions produced similar improvements in depression, quality of life, and a disease-specific measure but neither intervention produced improvements in physical function (six-minute walking distance). The third, and most recent study, that compared seven weeks of Qigong with wait-listed controls found significant improvements with Qigong, over usual care, in pain, depression, anxiety, quality of life, and sleep (13). These improvements were also significant (compared to baseline values) at an uncontrolled four-month follow-up (13).

Only two studies have addressed the merits of Tai Chi (an ancient Chinese martial art form). The first, an uncontrolled study, evaluated participants before and after they had received 12 one-hour sessions of Tai Chi. This study showed post–Tai Chi improvements in self-reported physical function, mood, pain, and fatigue (16). The second study, which used a stronger, randomized controlled design, evaluated the merits of 10 weeks of relaxation classes versus 10 weeks of education plus exercise (Tai Chi, postural training, strengthening, and stretching) (17). The education and exercise group had improvements versus the relaxation group on multiple measures at program end (four months postentry) but not at eight months (four months postprogram end). Further studies using a randomized controlled design with Tai Chi as a single intervention are required to establish the definitive benefits of Tai Chi.

PRACTICAL CONSIDERATIONS
Exercise-Specific Tips
Aerobic Exercise
Walking, low-impact fitness classes, and pool-based exercise programs are examples of aerobic exercises that are suitable for individuals with FM.

Pool-based aerobic exercise programs in warm (temperature $\geq$ 85°F) or therapeutic pools (temperature 91 to 98°F) are particularly suited as an *initial* means of exercise for those who are very deconditioned or for those who are afraid of postexercise pain, since water buoyancy limits the strain on weight-bearing joints and the warm water provides temporary relief from joint and muscle pain (18). Note that for a pool program to be aerobic, patients need to "move" in the water. Programs that involve standing or sitting with gentle stretching are not aerobic pool programs. In Europe, pool "therapy" also includes balneotherapy and thalassotherapy. Balneotherapy consists of immersion in warm water (usually natural spring water) with a high mineral content and is, therefore, not an example of pool "exercise." Thalassotherapy consists of exercise in seawater with/without other treatments. A recent, randomized controlled trial of 12 weeks of exercise in seawater versus 12 weeks of exercise in a regular pool found no additional benefit of sea versus regular water (both groups improved on pain, sleep, general health) with one exception: subjects who exercised in seawater had greater improvements in depression (19). However, the subjects in the seawater group were significantly more depressed at baseline than the control subjects and thus may have had more room for improvement.

To see gains in cardiorespiratory endurance, deconditioned individuals need to do aerobic exercise at least twice a week for a minimum of 20 minutes at a moderate intensity (64% of their maximum heart rate) (20). These guidelines apply to individuals with FM with one proviso: to minimize exercise-induced pain with aerobic exercise, they must start to exercise at a level *just below their capacity* and then *slowly increase* the duration and intensity of exercise until they reach the low end of moderate intensity [defined as heart rate while exercising of 220 minus individual's age (in years) × 64%]. For deconditioned individuals, heart rates compatible with moderate intensity can be achieved with low levels of exercise that should be gradually increased. Also note that if patients are on medications that control their heart rate, heart rates cannot be used to monitor exercise intensity. These patients can use the "talk test." In the talk test, exercise is not too intense if individuals can exercise and talk at the same time, without being short of breath. If exercise programs start off at too high an intensity, individuals with FM will either not be able to keep up with the rest of the group and/or will experience such significant postexercise pain that they will stop exercising. Individuals who are interested in joining general fitness programs should ask the instructor about the intensity of the classes and should be taught how to ease into an existing program (e.g., do less repetitions, exercise more slowly, take breaks). Sometimes fitness classes for seniors, with flexible rules on who can join the programs, are better options for individuals with FM as these programs may initially be less intense and then progress more slowly than other community-based fitness programs. Also, individuals should be forewarned that *aerobic exercise, even at appropriate intensity, will likely produce tolerable, short-term increases in postexercise pain and fatigue* that should dissipate within a few weeks of exercising.

Strengthening

Strengthening exercises should not work on the same muscle groups on consecutive days and there should be a rest between each set of a given exercise in a single exercise session. Strengthening should also be done at least twice a week. Finally, *no strengthening should be done to the maximum*, as this will cause postexercise pain. Subjects should also be cautioned that, like aerobic exercise, strengthening done at an appropriate intensity might cause temporary/tolerable increases in pain and fatigue that should abate with ongoing exercise.

To date, all strengthening-*only* studies have examined the benefits of isotonic exercise: exercise that is performed through a range of motion against constant resistance (e.g., when you extend your knee with a 3 lb weight on your ankle).

Some believe that isotonic exercise programs should not include *eccentric* exercise (where a muscle lengthens while contracting, for example, biceps lengthening while lowering a heavy object onto a table) as eccentric exercise can produce microtrauma in muscles and thereby increase postexercise pain (21). These same researchers suggest that even raising your arms overhead against gravity (eccentric work for biceps and deltoid muscles but also a common technique to increase the cardiovascular demands of low impact aerobics) should be avoided. However, we have found that exercise with arms overhead in aerobic classes is well tolerated if introduced slowly and performed in small bouts for limited periods of time.

Although no exercise trials have evaluated the merits of isometric exercise [the muscle contracts but the joint does not move (e.g., when you contract your quads with your knee already in extension)] in isolation, a recent article on pain processing employed isometric exercises as the experimental stimulus (22).

These investigators had individuals, with and without FM, sustain a hand grip for 90 seconds at 30% of maximum (an isometric exercise for finger flexors/extensors) while measuring self-reported heat pain and the threshold for mechanical pain, in both the exercising and nonexercising forearms at 30, 60, and 90 seconds. For individuals with FM, this submaximal grip increased self-reported heat pain at 60 and 90 seconds and lowered thresholds for mechanical pain at 30, 60, and 90 seconds, on both the exercising and nonexercising forearms. The opposite result was seen in control subjects. Thus for individuals with FM, submaximal isometric exercise on one side of their body *increased* pain on both sides of their body whereas the same exercise for control subjects *decreased* pain on both sides of their body.

Does this mean that isometric exercise should be avoided for individuals with FM? No. Clinically, individuals are instructed to do an isometric exercise for 5 to 10 seconds and not 30 to 90 seconds. Perhaps these exercise-induced increases in pain perception are only seen when exercising outside clinical parameters. Further, it is unclear whether similar results would be seen with *other* types of sustained or intense exercises (e.g., repeated isotonic exercise with maximal weight). If other kinds of exercises also caused pain on the nonexercising part of the body, this would suggest that intense or very sustained exercise, of any type, produces alterations in central pain processing in individuals with FM.

Stretching

Stretching should be included in all exercise programs as a warm-up activity and a cool-down activity. Stretching should be done to the point of mild resistance and not to the point of pain. Stretching or flexibility training may be beneficial as an *initial* means of exercise for those individuals who fear that exercise will produce intolerable increases in pain and fatigue. Stretching may also be therapeutic as an initial means of exercise for individuals who are very deconditioned and have impaired flexibility due to inactivity. However, individuals who begin with a stretching program should progress to aerobic or strengthening exercise programs.

Exercise Adherence

For exercise to be a viable treatment, individuals with FM need to exercise. Clinically, exercise adherence has two components. First, individuals need to be motivated to *begin* exercising. Then, they need to be motivated to *continue* to exercise.

Theoretically, once started, the act of exercise itself promotes ongoing exercise by enhancing self-efficacy (the belief that you can do a specific activity or behavior, in this case exercise). Motivational interviewing (MI) has also been suggested as a strategy to promote exercise initiation or ongoing adherence. In MI, a neutral interviewer helps an individual discuss the pros and cons of a new behavior (in this case, exercising) and how to overcome the barriers to beginning (or continuing) this behavior. There are two published accounts of the use of MI for promoting exercise in individuals with FM. In the first instance, the authors commented that MI was used to encourage individuals with FM to resume an exercise program (23). In the second instance, MI was used during an uncontrolled exercise trial to promote ongoing exercise adherence (24). In this uncontrolled trial, 19 individuals with FM received MI via five to six phone calls for the first 12 weeks of a home-based exercise program. Exercise adherence was measured after 12 and 30 weeks. Each subject in this trial was given an individualized exercise prescription of 5 to 10 minutes of exercise per day at moderate intensity (60% of age-adjusted maximal heart rate) to be done three times per week, with guidelines to increase the exercise duration per week by 1 to 2 minutes. These weekly expectations for exercise were low, as was the median reported exercise minutes per week at the end of 12 weeks (16 min/wk). Exercise activity was higher at 30 weeks (median, 32 min/wk). However, this study does not directly assess the effect of MI on exercise adherence because there was no control group.

Exercise Setting
Most studies have evaluated exercise programs in specialized settings (e.g., a hospital or a clinic). A few articles have been published on exercise programs in community facilities (11,17,25) or home-based exercise programs (26,27). Home-based exercise programs have the advantage of eliminating the need to find a suitable community program and can be tailored to the individual's exercise level and preferences but do not provide the social support of a group program. Individuals who do a home-based program need to be counseled that they will experience a short-term, tolerable increase in their pain for the first couple of weeks—otherwise they may conclude that exercise has made their FM "worse" and quit exercising.

Exercise is also Recommended for Children with FM
Although no exercise studies have been conducted on children with FM, exercise is recommended as an intervention for children with FM (28,29) because it is reasonable to think that the benefits of exercise would generalize to children with FM. Further, there is at least one published anecdote that physical activity and clinical improvement are significantly correlated. In this single report, children who reported greater physical activity at clinic follow-up also showed greater improvement in their clinical presentation (30).

FINAL REMARKS
Many studies have documented the benefits of aerobic exercises for individuals with FM. A much smaller number of recent studies also suggest that strengthening programs are helpful and well tolerated. Stretching should be included in every exercise program as a warm-up/cool-down activity, and may be used, as an initial means of exercise, but then individuals should progress to aerobic and/or strengthening programs. A significant barrier to exercise is that individuals with FM fear that exercise will increase pain, but exercise started at a level just below their physical capacity, and slowly increased, should produce only transient and tolerable increases in pain.

Given the current number of published studies on exercise for individuals with FM, future studies should use a randomized controlled design to assess the merits of exercise in this population. To be noteworthy, studies should also adequately describe the exercise intervention (type of exercise, exercise intensity/duration/frequency) and the clinical (disease duration, fitness/activity level, mood) and demographic characteristics (age, employment status) of the study sample.

REFERENCES

1. McCain G, Bell DA, Mai FM, et al. A controlled study of the effects of a supervised cardiovascular fitness training program on the manifestations of primary fibromyalgia. Arthritis Rheum 1988; 31:1135–1141.
2. BioMed Central. Health and Quality of Life Outcomes. Available at: http://www.hqlo.com/content/pdf/1477-7525-4-67.pdf. Accessed on September 2008.
3. Busch AJ, Barber KAR, Overend TJ, et al. Exercise for treating fibromyalgia syndrome. Cochrane Database Sys Rev 2007; (4): CD003786.
4. Valim V, Oliveira LM, Suda ÁL, et al. Peak oxygen uptake and ventilatory anaerobic threshold in fibromyalgia. J Rheumatol 2002; 29:353–357.
5. Wigers SH, Stiles TC, Vogel PA. Effects of aerobic exercise versus stress management treatment in fibromyalgia: a 4.5 year prospective study. Scand J Rheumatol 1996; 25:77–86.
6. Gowans SE, deHueck A, Voss S, et al. A randomized controlled clinical trial of education and physical training for individuals with fibromyalgia. Arthritis Care Res 1999; 12:120–128.
7. Gowans SE, deHueck A, Voss S, et al. Six-month and one-year follow-up of 23 weeks of aerobic exercise for individuals with fibromyalgia. Arthritis Rheum 2004; 51:890–898.
8. Mujika I, Padilla S. Cardiorespiratory and metabolic characteristics of detraining in humans. Med Sci Sports Exerc 2001; 33(3):413–421.
9. Hakkinen A, Hakkinen K, Hannonen P, et al. Strength training induced adaptations in neuromuscular function of premenopausal women with fibromyalgia: comparison with healthy women. Ann Rheum Dis 2001; 60:21–26.
10. Jones KD, Burckhardt CS, Clark SR, et al. A randomized controlled trial of muscle strengthening versus flexibility training in fibromyalgia. J Rheumatol 2002; 29: 1041–1048.
11. Kingsley JD, Panton LB, Toole T, et al. The effects of a 12-week strength-training program on strength and functionality in women with fibromyalgia. Arch Phys Med Rehabil 2005; 86:1713–1721.
12. Valkeinen H, Alen M, Hannonen P, et al. Changes in knee extension and flexion force, EMG and functional capacity during strength training in older females with fibromyalgia and healthy controls. Rheumatology 2004; 43:225–228.
13. Haak T, Scott B. The effect of qigong on fibromyalgia (FMS): a controlled randomized study. Disabil Rehabil 2008; 30(8):625–633.
14. Mannerkorpi K, Arndorw M. Efficacy and feasibility of a combination of body awareness therapy and qiqong in patients with fibromyalgia: a pilot study. J Rehabil Med 2004; 35:279–281.
15. Astin JA, Berman BM, Bausell B, et al. The efficacy of mindfulness meditation plus qigong movement therapy in the treatment of fibromyalgia: a randomized controlled trial. J Rheumatol 2003; 30:2257–2260.
16. Taggart HM, Arslanian CL, Bae S, et al. Effects of T'ai Chi exercise on fibromyalgia symptoms and health-related quality of life. Orthop Nurs 2003; 22:353–360.
17. Hammond A, Freeman K. Community patient education and exercise for people with fibromyalgia: a parallel group randomized controlled trial. Clin Rehabil 2006; 20:835–846.
18. Gowans SE, deHueck A. Pool exercise for individuals with fibromyalgia. Curr Opin Rheumatol 2007; 19(2):168–173.
19. de Andrade SC, de Carvalho RF, Soares AS, et al. Thalassotherapy for fibromyalgia: a randomized controlled trial comparing aquatic exercises in sea water and water pool. Rheumatol Int 2008; July 4 [Epub ahead of print].
20. American College of Sports Medicine. ACSM's Guidelines for Exercise Testing and Prescription. 7th ed. Baltimore: Lippincott, Williams and Wilkins, 2006.
21. Clark SR, Jones KD, Burckhardt CS, et al. Exercise for patients with fibromyalgia: risks versus benefits. Curr Rheumatol Rep 2001; 3:135–146.
22. Staud R, Robinson ME, Price DD. Isometric exercise has opposite effects on central pain mechanisms in fibromyalgia patients compared to normal controls. Pain 2005; 118:176–184.

23. Jones KD, Burckhardt CS, Bennet JA. Motivational interviewing may encourage exercise in persons with fibromyalgia by enhancing self-efficacy. Arthritis Rheum 2004; 51:864–867.
24. Ang D, Kesavalu R, Lydon JR. Exercise-based motivational interviewing for female patients with fibromyalgia: a case series. Clin Rheumatol 2007; 26:1843–1849.
25. Dawson KA, Tiidus PM, Pierrynowski M, et al. Evaluation of a community-based exercise program for diminishing symptoms of fibromyalgia. Physiother Can 2003; 55:17–22.
26. DaCosta DD, Abrahamawicz M, Lowensheyn I, et al. A randomized clinical trial of an individualized home-based exercise programme for women with fibromyalgia. Rheumatology 2005; 44:1422–1427.
27. Schacter CL, Busch AJ, Peloso PM, et al. Effects of short versus long bouts of aerobic exercise in sedentary women with fibromyalgia: a randomized controlled trial. Phys Ther 2003; 83:340–358.
28. Burckhardt C, Goldenberg D, Crofford L, et al. Guideline for the Management of Pain in Adults and Children with Fibromyalgia Syndrome. Glenview, IL: American Pain Society, 2005.
29. Anthony KK, Schanberg LE. Assessment and management of pain syndromes and arthritis pain in children and adolescents. Rheum Dis Clin North Am 2007; 33:625–660.
30. Gedalia A, Garcia CO, Molina JF, et al. Fibromyalgia syndrome: experience in a pediatric rheumatology clinic. Clin Exp Rheumatol 2000; 18(3):415–419.

8 Motivating Behavioral Change in Fibromyalgia

David A. Williams
Chronic Pain and Fatigue Research Center, and Department of Anesthesiology,
Medicine, Psychiatry, and Psychology, University of Michigan, Ann Arbor,
Michigan, U.S.A.

Marissa L. Marshak
Clinical Social Worker, Ann Arbor, Michigan, U.S.A.

INTRODUCTION

Fibromyalgia (FM) is an extreme manifestation of chronic widespread pain (CWP) with a prevalence of 2% in the general population (1). Clinically, individuals with FM present with a variety of symptoms including widespread pain, fatigue, tenderness, sleep disturbance, decrements in physical functioning, and disruptions in psychological functioning (e.g., memory problems, concentration difficulties, diminished mental clarity, mood disturbances, and lack of well-being) (2–5). FM occurs more frequently in females and the comorbid overlap of FM with related functional disorders [e.g., temporomandibular disorder (TMD), irritable bowel syndrome (IBS), chronic fatigue syndrome (CFS)] is extremely high (6,7). Triggering of FM requires a genetic predisposition coupled with environmental stressors (8–13). The maintenance of FM symptoms over time appears related to centrally mediated amplification of the processes integrating sensory, cognitive, and affective information, dysfunction in endogenous noxious inhibitory systems, sleep disturbance, and dysautonomia (14–18). Thus, it is likely that there are multiple dysregulated pathways by which a given individual can develop the clinical picture qualifying for the diagnosis of FM.

Currently there is strong evidence supporting the benefits of several pharmacological agents, aerobic exercise, and specific cognitive and behavioral lifestyle adaptations for the management of FM (19). While no single intervention appears to address all aspects of well-being for FM, combinations of these interventions appear to offer benefits to individuals who are motivated to undertake the lifestyle adaptations associated with this combination of treatments (20).

DUALLY FOCUSED INTERVENTIONS FOR FM

Dually focused interventions combine pharmacological agents (e.g., aimed at pain reduction) with behavioral change (e.g., aimed at improved functional status). While pain is the cardinal symptom of FM, many other symptoms or complaints accompany this diagnosis (21,22). While some of these symptoms emanate from triggering factors, other symptoms may result from having persistent pain. For example, prolonged resting in response to pain may diminish the perception of pain in the short term, but lead to muscular deconditioning in the long term. Once deconditioned, a potent pain reliever will be incapable of restoring functional status as a monotherapy. Dually focused interventions recognize the important interplay between the pharmacological benefits of pain relief and the essential behavioral work that is needed to restore function. In the case of FM, pain relief is often incomplete so the behavioral work must focus on adaptation and lifestyle adjustment rather than on complete restoration of premorbid function.

COGNITIVE BEHAVIORAL THERAPY

Cognitive behavioral therapy (CBT) has the strongest evidence-base supporting its use in an intervention for making life-style adaptations in individuals with FM (19,23). CBT has its origins within the traditional psychotherapy literature but has been modified for applications with many medical conditions [e.g., coronary disease (24), cancer survival (25), and chronic pain (26)]. While the specific skills used in each application of CBT differ depending on the needs of the condition, the techniques used to change behavior are based on principles of classical and operant conditioning (e.g., extinction, positive and negative reinforcement, shaping, prompts), and observational learning (27,28). The techniques used to produce cognitive changes are based largely on the development of problem-solving skills and principles of attributional change (29,30).

In a review of 25 CBT trials for chronic pain, this class of intervention was credited with producing significant improvements in pain and function generally (31). More specifically, CBT has demonstrated efficacy for rheumatological conditions such as osteoarthritis (OA) and rheumatoid arthritis (RA) (32–34), and in the case of FM, CBT may have its greatest impact on the domain of improving functional status (23,35).

CBT Skill Sets Common to FM

CBT interventions typically include three phases: (*i*) an educational phase—in which patients are familiarized with a model for understanding their pain and the role that individuals can play in the management of the condition (e.g., the biopsychosocial model), (*ii*) a skills-training phase—in which training is provided in a variety of cognitive and behavioral skills useful for managing pain and improving function (e.g., relaxation training, activity pacing), and (*iii*) an application phase—in which patients learn to apply their skills in progressively more challenging real-life situations (36). Each application of CBT for FM needs to be tailored to the needs of the patient, and a clear treatment target needs to be agreed upon by both the therapist and the patient (e.g., focus on pain, function, sleep, etc.). The most common behavioral changes attempted through CBT for FM include the following: (*i*) adoption of the relaxation response into daily practice, (*ii*) adoption of graded activation and pleasant activity scheduling as a means of improving functional status, (*iii*) behavioral methods to improve sleep and cognition, (*iv*) problem-solving and cognitive-restructuring techniques to increase productivity and reduce stress, and (*v*) communication skills to facilitate more beneficial relationships between patients and physicians, family members, and friends.

The Relaxation Response

The relaxation response is thought to be a highly beneficial nonpharmacological method of reducing pain through diminished autonomic arousal (37). The body will naturally relax when individuals perceive the absence of threat or stressful environmental demands. Pain, however, is a persistent stressor precluding opportunities to perceive safety and naturally evoke physiological relaxation. Patients with chronic pain must therefore learn to trigger relaxation under their own conscious control.

The relaxation response is a physiologically based learned response that involves quieting physiological activity (e.g., muscle tension, heart rate, and breathing) through active and focused mental effort. Learning the response requires the individual to practice the techniques repeatedly until his or her body acquires the desired response. While there is no consensus as to the best method of teaching the relaxation response (e.g., progressive muscle relaxation, visual imagery, hypnosis, biofeedback), all appear to be useful modalities for learning this response.

In the case of FM, early attempts to use the relaxation response for pain reduction focused on muscular relaxation (e.g., using EMG in biofeedback and/ or progressive muscle relaxation) were based on early notions regarding the etiology of FM (i.e., it was assumed that the pain of FM was related to muscle spasms or muscle tightness). With increased understanding, the focus of relaxation-based treatments shifted from the peripheral muscle to central mechanisms. Thus it is likely that the benefits of the relaxation response stem more from its systemic calming than from reduction of tension in any specific muscle.

Graded Activation and Pleasant Activity Scheduling

While pain is often the presenting symptom in FM, perhaps the most challenging aspect of FM is dealing with fatigue and improving physical functional status (21,35). For many, fatigue impairs multiple aspects of life including work productivity, social engagement, and personal hobbies/pleasant activities. Most individuals with FM will attempt to pace their activities, placing essential tasks before personal pleasures. While this strategy benefits employers, day after day of denying personal pleasures can have devastating effects on mood and motivation. Denial of pleasurable activities augments pain and further reduces function.

Taking time to engage in pleasant activities should not be viewed as an excessive selfish indulgence. Quite the contrary, enjoyment of pleasant activities is a natural way to elevate mood (38) and invites confidence in ones' body to function at a higher level. This behavioral change encourages scheduling pleasant activities into ones' day with the same priority as a meeting, a doctor's appointment, or a deadline. Scheduling is far more preferable to spontaneity given spontaneity may never occur, or if it does, may occur at a time when the patient is vulnerable to overdoing and risking increased pain.

In order to avoid overdoing, pleasant activity scheduling is often paired with skills in graded activation. Many patients unwittingly worsen pain on "good days" by doing more than personal limitations allow. This overactivity is followed by several "bad days" of symptom flares. An intermittent burst of activity followed by increased pain is a source of frustration for patients as the ability to plan and predict function becomes limited. Graded activation is a method of pacing which can improve physical functioning while minimizing the likelihood of pain flare-ups. This approach has been successfully applied with low back pain populations (39), rheumatological populations (40), and in patients having chronic fatigue syndrome (41). The key to this strategy is to limit activities based on time rather than on patients' subjective experience of pain or task completion. Active time can be as short as several minutes or as long as several hours depending on what the patient can initially tolerate without exacerbation. Once the patient and the therapist agree on a time-based activity program, subsequent goals for steadily increasing the amount of time spent on specified targeted behaviors can proceed. Time-based pacing can be used as a complimentary skill to help ensure the long-term adoption of exercise regimens, work-related activities, and pleasant activities such as social outings and sports activities.

Behavioral Methods for Improving Sleep and Cognition

Individuals with FM have a number of problems related to getting a good night's sleep including difficulty falling asleep, being awakened by pain or discomfort, or if able to fall asleep, will awaken feeling unrefreshed and unrestored. There exist a number of behavioral strategies that, if used regularly, can help individuals get needed restorative sleep with additional benefits in improved mood, better management of pain, less fatigue, and improved mental clarity (42). Some of these skills focus on timing strategies (e.g., having regular sleep routines), sleep behaviors (e.g., attempting to sleep only when in need of sleep), and behavioral avoidance of stimulating activities before bed such as emotionally charged conversations, watching action movies, or consuming nicotine or caffeine. CBT targeting sleep appears to have a direct impact on pain symptoms and on functional interference resulting from nonrestorative sleep (43–45). Like the relaxation response, behavioral strategies for improving sleep are physiological self-regulation skills that require repeated practice and consistency to train the body to respond in the desired manner under conscious control.

Often individuals with FM will report diminished cognitive function. Known in the patient community as "fibro-fog," this form of dyscognition is experienced as involving difficulties with concentration and attention, memory, and mental clarity. The cause of dyscognition associated with FM is not well understood but is likely to be associated with the lack of restorative sleep architecture and the distracting nature of persistent pain on information processing (46,47). Behavioral approaches such as the relaxation response for pain and behavioral approaches to improve sleep are likely to benefit fibro-fog.

Problem-Solving Strategies and Cognitive Restructuring

Individuals with FM face interpersonal and functional challenges that do not even cross the minds of healthy individuals. The daily barrage of seemingly novel and unsolvable challenges adds to the fatigue and burden of the individual with FM. Programmatic problem-solving strategies that help to break large problems down into solvable pieces can be taught to patients (48,49). What is taught in therapy is a strategy for solving problems rather than specific solutions; thus patients learn a strategy that can be carried into the future as new problems arise. When applied successfully, patients learn to overcome barriers and attain a greater sense of control over the process of adapting to a chronic illness.

Solutions to problems often reflect beliefs about the nature of the problem and beliefs about one's personal ability to effectively execute solutions. Strong convictions in ones' helplessness, the futility of trying to control illness, or the inability to contribute meaningfully to others are examples of learned automatic thinking patterns that impede successful adaptation. Cognitive restructuring (50) is a cognitive skill that challenges the rationality of automatic thoughts such as those above and seeks to instill alternative thinking that promotes greater function and well-being. This skill is often confused with "positive thinking," which can be perceived as ingenuine and unrealistic if the suggested thinking patterns fall too far outside the perceived reality of the patient with pain. Cognitive restructuring invites patients to explore the origin of learned automatic thinking processes that promote maladaptive behavior in response to pain. Fortunately, with practice, new thinking patterns can replace old ones that are more consistent with well-being and functioning even with the discomforts associated with FM.

Communication Skills
Individuals with FM frequently report unsatisfying visits with their physicians stemming from the perception that an exchange of information sufficient for the proper treatment of FM did not occur. The cause of this insufficient exchange is multifaceted including such factors as too little time, becoming disorganized and forgetting to mention all that was important, physicians having their own agenda of questions, and interpersonal factors such as desire to please the physician, being afraid of the physician, etc.

Regardless of the cause, the patient needs to feel adequately understood by the clinician providing care. The patient may need to actively participate in making this happen. While it is unlikely that the patient will be able change the behavior of the clinician, there are many behavioral strategies that can be used by the patient to improve doctor-patient communication. Similarly, family members need to understand what they can do to be most helpful to the patient. A common mistake of family members is to remove all responsibility from the patient in order to facilitate rest and remove stress. This is often the wrong approach, as individuals with FM need to be able to engage in activities that empower them to feel efficacious and productive. Communicating with family and friends about how best to support such efforts can require tact and good bit of assertiveness.

Assertive communication skills training (51,52) represents a skill set that is easily communicated to individuals but is best implemented with consistent practice or role playing with a therapist. Typically, a bit of trial and error helps to refine ones' personal strengths in being appropriately assertive.

Delivery of CBT
CBT is commonly delivered in either a 1:1 format between a trained therapist and a single patient or with a therapist in a group setting. Currently, both formats appear to be effective with anecdotal clinical experience, suggesting added benefit from the social exchange that occurs between patients in well-conducted group therapy. While optimally delivered in either of these formats with a doctoral level therapist possessing postdoctoral training in pain management or behavioral medicine, such professionals are not easily accessible to the average primary care practitioner. Alternatives to traditional CBT delivery methods are finding their way into clinical practice. One example is the delivery

of coping skills training over the telephone (53). In this application, many of the cognitive and behavioral skills of CBT are taught to patients by either doctoral level or allied health staff members. In studies with patients having RA, similar cognitive and behavioral skills have been taught and supported by lay coaches (54). Our group at the University of Michigan has adapted many of the CBT-supported skills useful for FM and developed static educational websites, workbooks, and CD media that can be used for self-management in highly motivated individuals or as a companion to more traditional face-to-face CBT with a licensed therapist.

Barriers Implementing Behavioral Changes in FM

The behavioral changes just described are not intuitive. In fact, some are contrary to ones' natural inclinations. For example, it is not natural to relax when one's body perceives a threat such as pain; it is not natural to remain active (even for a brief time) when resting seems to relieve pain; and it is more natural to isolate oneself when feeling pain than to engage in pleasant and/or social activities. Thus, many of the behaviors that are intuitive for the management of acute pain are actually quite different from the behaviors found to be adaptive for the long-term management of chronic pain. This fact may seem puzzling at first if one assumes that chronic pain is simply acute pain that lasts too long. The truth is, chronic pain is far more complex than acute pain. While acute pain serves a protective bodily function and is a healthy physiological response to danger, chronic pain is a disorder and requires its own therapeutic approach (i.e., dually focused interventions). Thus, the behavioral changes used for long-term management of chronic pain must be explained to both patients and clinicians as there is no universal understanding of this important distinction.

For some individuals, simply understanding what to do will be sufficiently motivating to lead them to adopt meaningful behavioral changes. For others, simple education will be insufficiently motivating or insufficiently structured to support behavioral change over the long term. For clinicians to successfully implement both aspects of dually focused treatment in the broad array of individuals presenting with FM, it is helpful to have a stronger understanding of the elements underlining motivation.

THEORIES OF MOTIVATION

Over the past century, the field of psychology has generated numerous theories on motivation as it pertains to behavioral control. These theories address a continuum of behavior from highly specialized functions (thought to be hard-wired and requiring little learning) to more general purpose behavioral control mechanisms.

Biological Motives and Primary Affects

Some motives help guide behavior toward maintaining internal homeostasis or adapting to changing environmental conditions for the survival of the organism. For example, reflexes are innate biological behavioral control mechanisms that govern highly specific behaviors (e.g., salivation in response to food). In the case of reflexes, the relevant behaviors are fixed behaviors and do not require learning.

Primary affect is tied closely to the internal regulation of the organism; it is an innate behavioral control mechanism and is essentially unlearned. Unlike biological motives that subserve highly specific biological functions (e.g., temperature regulation, breathing, nourishment, etc), primary affect varies depending on the conditions under which it is experienced and does not evoke specific behavioral responses. Primary affect includes happiness, sadness, fear, anger, surprise, interest, shame, and disgust/contempt (55,56). Like biological drives when negative primary affect is experienced, the individual is motivated to reduce this experience through behavioral responses.

Primary drives are innate behavior control mechanisms triggered by internal deprivation of bodily tissue. Unlike reflexes however, the behavioral response to tissue deprivation is nonspecific and can take alternative forms as long as the evoked behaviors eventually lead to rectifying the deprivation. For example, natural tissue needs can result from deprivation of air, water, food, sleep, etc., setting into motion behavior control mechanisms aimed at reducing these drives. Behaviors leading to successful drive reduction (i.e., placing an organism back into a stable biological state) can be highly reinforcing; thus these behavioral patterns are likely to be chosen again when similar needs arise. One could state that the drive-reducing qualities of engaging in such behaviors are what motivate the decision to engage in a specific behavior. That is, individuals are motivated to perform behaviors that satisfy drives.

Pain is a biological state for which there is a strong drive for its reduction. Since drives are nonspecific motivators of behavior, there are many behaviors that could potentially reduce this drive (e.g., taking a narcotic, distracting oneself, avoiding the painful stimulus, resting, etc.). As already stated, individuals with chronic pain often rely on methods of reducing discomfort from acute pain, which can be maladaptive in the context of chronic pain and must be unlearned or modified.

Acquired Drives

Not all drives motivate behaviors that subserve the immediate biological survival of the organism. For example, some individuals are motivated toward personal achievement, affiliation with others, personal power, or accumulation of money. Whereas biological drives are innate and the behaviors used to satisfy the drive is learned, acquired drives form in such a way that both the satisfying behaviors and the value of the goal (i.e., the basis of the drive) must be learned. Once learned however, acquired drives act just like biological drives in terms of their ability to evoke and reinforce specific behaviors when the drives are reduced and satisfied. Unlike biological drives that rarely lose their salience for the individual, the value of acquired drives can be more variable. For example, an individual may value money for most of his or her life only to change to valuing personal time over money in later life. Acquired drives have been extensively studied and tend to fall into three categories: achievement competence, affiliation attachment, and power dominance (57,58).

Effectance Motivation

Why would humans explore their environment if they were not trying to quiet a biological drive? What biological drive is being satisfied by seeking sensory stimulation in the form of going to a movie or playing a video game? Effectance motivation refers to an innate need to experience competence in dealing with the environment. The drive, therefore, is to experience effectance; any behaviors that satisfy that need get reinforced and are more likely to be repeated. The need to effectively manipulate the environment is thought to underlie play in children (and adults), as well as being the motivational force associated with advanced cognitive development (59). Individuals with pain often have energy only to satisfy the most immediate and primary of needs leaving innate drives for effectance, play, and cognitive development unmet.

THE CONCEPTS OF INTRINSIC AND EXTRINSIC MOTIVATION

The very idea that one person wants to motivate another to perform specific behaviors congers up the dynamics of interpersonal relationships and the fact that reinforcers of behavior (i.e., motivators) can reside both within the individual (i.e., intrinsic motivation) or with another person (i.e., extrinsic motivation).

Intrinsic Motivation

Intrinsic motivation refers to behavioral control mechanisms associated with drive-reducing behaviors falling completely under the control of the individual. Thus, personal control (or the perception/belief that one has personal control) is an important concept associated with intrinsic motivation (60–63). Generally, perceived personal control over biological and environmental events positively impacts psychological and behavioral functioning. For example, intrinsic motivation has been associated with greater achievement and enjoyment in educational settings (64), greater satisfaction and productivity in work settings (65,66), and improved adherence and better outcomes in medical settings (67).

Extrinsic Motivation and Reward

Extrinsic motivation is a special case of motivation that involves the concept of a reward. While many reinforcers of behavior are intrinsic, reward is unique in that its delivery is under the control of another individual or part of the environment external to the individual. For a reward to be motivating, the reward must have value in satisfying a need and must be perceived as being beyond the ability of the individual to acquire on his or her own. For example, a child will become hungry and desire food. Perceiving an inability to acquire food himself or herself, the child will turn to an adult to provide the food. The adult has the choice of giving the food freely or requiring some behavior (e.g., hand washing, cleaning up the room) before offering the reward. Since hunger is a strong biological drive, the child is likely to be highly motivated to perform whatever behaviors are necessary to receive food and satisfy the biological drive. As is obvious, extrinsic motivation can be quite powerful and can be used either altruistically or to the detriment of well-being in the form of coercion (68).

Important to the concept of extrinsic motivation is an interpersonal dynamic involving a power differential between the individual with the need (i.e., the person whose behavior is being shaped) and the individual holding the reward (i.e., the person who wants to motivate behavioral change). This power differential will remain intact so long as (*i*) a need persists and (*ii*) individuals with the need continue to perceive that they are incapable of satisfying the need on their own. For example, in the case of the hungry child, the child is truly dependent on adults; in other circumstances, the power differential is not inherent but willingly adopted. In the latter circumstances, the power differential can be dissolved should there be a breach of trust or other interpersonal transgression that overshadows the benefit of maintaining the dependent relationship associated with receiving the reward. Employment relationships serve as an example where productivity for pay is maintained so long as there is satisfaction and respect for the leadership. Therapeutic relationships are another example of a voluntary power differential where patients turn to clinicians for help so long as there is the perception that their condition is understood and that they are being appropriately cared for and respected as patients.

MOTIVATION IN MEDICAL SETTINGS

Traditionally, the biomedical model has emphasized interventions that require a clinician to produce improvements (e.g., dispensing medications, massages, surgery, nerve blocks, etc.). Thus, a relationship involving a power differential is common to most biomedical approaches for pain control. In order for pain to diminish (i.e., a reward), the patient must form and then follow the rules of a relationship with a clinician (i.e., the holder of the intervention). Under this model, direct pain relief comes from actions performed by the clinician and not by the patient, thus making the clinician essential to drive reduction. The patients' role in drive reduction is indirect and limited to getting the physician to perform his or her behaviors that lead to drive reduction. Thus the patient behaviors that get reinforced are those that maximize patients' abilities to extract drive-reducing rewards from clinicians (i.e., an extrinsic model of motivation). Under the biomedical model, patients are likely to develop a strong attachment to the holder of the reward. With acute pain, dependence on the clinician lasts only so long as the drive exists and the value of the reward naturally diminishes with the resolution of the pain. In chronic pain, however, the drive state does not resolve by definition, thus laying the foundation for a protracted, dependent relationship.

CBT, on the other hand, differs from the biomedical model in that by design it is a short-term intervention for a long-term problem that bypasses the use of reward. While CBT is based on learning and heavily relies on reinforcement to promote behavioral change, it does so without the use of reward. In CBT, the therapist does not want patients to become dependent on the therapist for making needed lifestyle changes, but rather to have patients experience reinforcement intrinsically by seeing and experiencing connections between personal effort and successful management of FM (69). Key to establishing intrinsic motivation for behavioral change is the establishment of beliefs in personal control through goal setting and symptom monitoring.

Beliefs in Personal Control

Beliefs in personal control are thought to evolve from multiple learning experiences where personal effort is perceived to affect outcomes. The perception of personal control has been termed an "internal" locus of control. Alternatively, an "external" locus of control is learned when outcomes are perceived as occurring outside of personal control.

Beliefs in locus of control that are specific to matters of health have been termed health locus of control beliefs (HLOC) (70) and can include either internal beliefs (i.e., personal control over health) or beliefs in external control (e.g., powerful doctors or chance happenings). Studies of preventive healthcare behaviors have found that stronger beliefs in internal locus are associated with improved ability to stop smoking (71,72), greater weight loss (73,74), adherence to birth control regimens (75), and receiving preventive inoculations (76). Findings in the preventive healthcare arena parallel those from education where students with an internal locus of control tended to show better academic achievement, studied longer, and put forth greater personal effort for academic achievement (77,78). In general, the belief in internal locus of control reflects a learned expectation that personal effort will result in a predictable outcome that can satisfy a drive to effectively address biologically or environmentally driven needs.

Locus of control for pain refers to patients' perceptions about their personal ability to control pain. Most patients with FM generally have a more external locus of control than other chronic pain conditions (79–81). This is perhaps due to a history of unsuccessful attempts to apply intuitive yet flawed acute pain management approaches to a chronic pain condition resulting in failure. Repeated failures to personally influence the pain of FM through rest and other acute pain strategies is likely to lay the foundation for the development of an external locus of control and the perceived need to depend on others for help. Fortunately, such learning can be supplanted by new learned relationships between personal effort and the management of FM. Goal setting and symptom monitoring are two tools that greatly facilitate insight leading to a stronger belief in internal locus of control.

Studies of patients with chronic pain and rheumatological conditions support the ability of individuals with chronic pain to benefit from strengthening their beliefs in internal locus of control. An internal locus for pain control has been repeatedly associated with lower levels of physical and psychological symptoms and better response to therapy (82–91). In FM, internal locus of control has been associated with better affect, reduced symptom severity, less disability in both upper and lower extremity functions, and generally improved levels of functional status in FM (81). Currently, several randomized controlled trials are evaluating the benefits of improving internal locus of control as a means of motivating lasting lifestyle modifications for FM (92,93).

Stages of Change
Knowing what to change and how to do it is insufficient for ensuring that behavioral change will occur. Similarly improving internal locus of control by identifying linkages between personal effort and symptom reduction relies on patients actually taking the first steps toward self-management. Sometimes individuals are simply not ready to adopt new behaviors and take on the personal responsibility of self-management.

The transtheoretical model conjectures that changes in behaviors evolve through six stages of change: precontemplation, contemplation, preparation, action, maintenance, and termination (94,95). Early uses of "Stages of Change" model were associated with behavioral attempts to quit smoking. For example, an individual may be in the contemplation stage if he or she desires to quit smoking, but has not sought the necessary resources to make the actual behavioral change(s). Alternatively, an individual who has actively sought resources and made some attempts to quit would be considered to be in the action stage. Although these stages are represented in a linear format, there is a "relapse" stage, which can revert an individual back any number of stages. Kerns et al. (96) have translated the stages of change to be used with chronic pain conditions and suggest that there are specific characteristics and techniques associated with each stage that can help motivate individuals with chronic pain to make necessary behavioral changes.

To help assess readiness to make behavioral adaptations, Kerns developed the Pain Stages of Change Questionnaire (PSOCQ) (96). As primary care physicians may not be as comfortable in developing a behavioral treatment regimen as they are in developing a pharmacological one, this instrument has utility in treatment planning. The concept of stages of change also serves as a useful educational tool for helping patients understand the need for their personal involvement in FM management. The Stages of Change model is not pejorative or blaming those who are not ready to make behavioral changes; rather it acknowledges that each individual has his or her own timeframe and process for determining readiness to adopt new behaviors.

Motivational Interviewing

Acknowledging that individuals have different stages of readiness to make behavioral adaptations does not mean that the clinician is without resources for accelerating his or her patients along their paths. Motivational interviewing (MI) is one such resource (97). Many MI techniques address issues associated with the contemplative stages of change as they focus on identifying what behavioral changes need to be made. As individuals explore options, there is an opportunity to help individuals design or plan movements toward the "action" stages. MI has been best applied in changing high-risk health behaviors where clinicians can leverage "teachable moments." For example, a young male may have been thinking about wearing a motorcycle helmet but never bought one. A few well-timed motivational comments from an astute clinician in the emergency room where his friend is being treated for head injuries could accelerate his adopting helmet-wearing behavior in the future.

Often individuals fail to make behavioral changes until the need for such smacks them in the face. A frequent story from cardiac rehabilitation is that of the patient who talks about wanting to adopt a healthier lifestyle but was not sufficiently motivated until after the heart attack. Obviously, it would be better if teachable moments could be identified before an acute crisis.

The power of a teachable moment stems from the ability to capitalize on a real-life event (not a hypothetical risk factor) where the patient is able to see linkages between the problem and behaviors that can fall under the patient's personal control to correct or prevent. Given these opportune "moments" are so powerful, clinicians are encouraged to search for them across many conditions so as to persuade patients to adopt healthy behaviors generally (98). In an office visit, by being aware of the potential for teachable moments, the clinician can have great impact in supporting movement toward meaningful long-term changes in lifestyle without taking too much time away from resolving the presenting problem.

In the case of FM, the clinician will need to know and listen to the patient carefully in order to identify teachable moments. Teachable moments are likely to be attendant to situations leading to pain flares (e.g., over doing when deconditioned), sadness and isolation, work avoidance, stress, and fatigue. MI has been shown to be a useful method for encouraging individuals with FM in the initiation and maintenance of exercise regimens even when pain was perceived as being a barrier (97). In this instance, MI was successful in eliciting quick, long-term results. It should be remembered, however, that MI is a method for accelerating movement toward the long-term adoption of healthy behaviors and is best used in conjunction with more comprehensive, evidenced-based behavioral change programs like CBT.

CONCLUSION
As the primary care physician adopts a frontline stance in the care of individuals with FM, he or she will need both pharmacological and behavioral tools to help manage this condition. Given that dually focused interventions for FM are likely to continue to be the basis on which the most comprehensive improvements in FM occur, motivating patients to adopt complex multicomponent changes in lifestyle will be essential. Approaches such as CBT, knowledge of stages of change, MI and teachable moments, and the use of symptom monitoring and goal setting are valuable tools toward this end. The primary care physician will be most successful when he or she enables patients to see relationships between their own personal actions and improvements in their condition. The generation of a strong internal locus of control in patients allows them to become partners with the clinician in the management of FM over the long term.

ACKNOWLEDGMENT
Supported in part by grant numbers R01-AR050044 (NIAMS/NIH), AR053207 (NIAMS/NIH), U01AR55069 (NIAMS/NIH), and DAMD 17-00-2-0018 (Department of Defense).

REFERENCES
1. Wolfe F, Ross K, Anderson J, et al. The prevalence and characteristics of fibromyalgia in the general population. Arthritis Rheum 1995; 38(1):19–28.
2. Yunus MB. Symptoms and signs of fibromyalgia syndrome: an overview. In: Wallace DJ, Clauw DJ, eds. Fibromyalgia and Other Central Pain Syndromes. Philadelphia, PA: Lippincott Williams & Wilkins, 2005:125–132.
3. Wolfe F, Hawley DJ. Psychosocial factors and the fibromyalgia syndrome. Z Rheumatol 1998; 57(suppl 2):88–91.
4. Forseth KO, Gran JT. Management of fibromyalgia: what are the best treatment choices? Drugs 2002; 62(4):577–592.
5. Mease PJ, Clauw DJ, Arnold LM, et al. Fibromyalgia syndrome. J Rheumatol 2005; 32(11):2270–2277.
6. Clauw DJ, Chrousos GP. Chronic pain and fatigue syndromes: overlapping clinical and neuroendocrine features and potential pathogenic mechanisms. Neuroimmunomodulation 1997; 4(3):134–153.
7. Aaron LA, Burke MM, Buchwald D. Overlapping conditions among patients with chronic fatigue syndrome, fibromyalgia, and temporomandibular disorder. Arch Intern Med 2000; 160(2):221–227.
8. Buskila D, Neumann L, Vaisberg G, et al. Increased rates of fibromyalgia following cervical spine injury. A controlled study of 161 cases of traumatic injury [see comments]. Arthritis Rheum 1997; 40(3):446–452.

9. Waylonis GW, Perkins RH. Post-traumatic fibromyalgia. A long-term follow-up. Am J Phys Med Rehabil 1994; 73(6):403–412.
10. Goldenberg DL. Fibromyalgia and its relation to chronic fatigue syndrome, viral illness and immune abnormalities. J Rheumatol Suppl 1989; 19:91–93.
11. Culclasure TF, Enzenauer RJ, West SG. Post-traumatic stress disorder presenting as fibromyalgia. Am J Med 1993; 94(5):548–549.
12. Hazlett RL, Haynes SN. Fibromyalgia: a time-series analysis of the stressor-physical symptom association. J Behav Med 1992; 15(6):541–558.
13. Dailey PA, Bishop GD, Russell IJ, et al. Psychological stress and the fibrositis/ fibromyalgia syndrome. J Rheumatol 1990; 17(10):1380–1385.
14. Moldofsky H. Sleep and pain. Sleep Med Rev 2001; 5(5):385–396.
15. Moldofsky H. Sleep, neuroimmune and neuroendocrine functions in fibromyalgia and chronic fatigue syndrome. Adv Neuroimmunol 1995; 5(1):39–56.
16. Martinez-Lavin M, Hermosillo AG, Rosas M, et al. Circadian studies of autonomic nervous balance in patients with fibromyalgia: a heart rate variability analysis. Arthritis Rheum 1998; 41(11):1966–1971.
17. Martinez-Lavin M. Dysfunction of the autonomic nervous system in chronic pain syndromes. In: Wallace DJ, Clauw DJ, eds. Fibromyalgia and Other Central Pain Syndromes. Philadelphia: Lippincott Williams and Wilkins, 2005:81–88.
18. Williams DA, Gracely RH. Biology and therapy of fibromyalgia. Functional magnetic resonance imaging findings in fibromyalgia. Arthritis Res Ther 2006; 8(6):224.
19. Goldenberg DL, Burckhardt C, Crofford L. Management of fibromyalgia syndrome. JAMA 2004; 292(19):2388–2395.
20. Williams DA. Psychological and behavioral therapies in fibromyagia and related syndromes. Best Pract Res Clin Rheumatol 2003; 17(4):649–665.
21. Bennett RM, Jones J, Turk DC, et al. An internet survey of 2,596 people with fibro-myalgia. BMC Musculoskelet Disord 2007; 8:27.
22. Mease P, Arnold LM, Bennett R, et al. Fibromyalgia syndrome. J Rheumatol 2007; 34 (6):1415–1425.
23. Williams DA, Cary MA, Groner KH, et al. Improving physical functional status in patients with fibromyalgia: a brief cognitive behavioral intervention. J Rheumatol 2002; 29(6):1280–1286.
24. Blumenthal JA, Jiang W, Babyak MA, et al. Stress management and exercise training in cardiac patients with myocardial ischemia. Effects on prognosis and evaluation of mechanisms. Arch Intern Med 1997; 157(19):2213–2223.
25. Fawzy FI, Fawzy NW, Arndt LA, et al. Critical review of psychosocial interventions in cancer care. Arch Gen Psychiatry 1995; 52(2):100–113.
26. Turk DC. Biopsychosocial perspective on chronic pain. In: Gatchel RJ, Turk DC, eds. Psychological Approaches to Pain Management: A Practitioner's Handbook. New York: Guilford Press, 1996:3–32.
27. Craighead LW, Craighead WE, Kazdin AE, et al. Cognitive and Behavioral Inter-ventions: An Empiracle Approach to Mental Health Problems. Boston: Allyn and Bacon, 1994.
28. Keefe FJ, Gil KM, Rose SC. Behavioral approaches in the multidisciplinary management of chronic pain: programs and issues. Clin Psychol Rev 1986; 6:87–113.
29. Sacco WP, Beck AT. Cognitive therapy of depression. In: Beckham EE, Leber WR, eds. Handbook of Depression: Treatment, Assessment, and Research. Homewood: Dorsey Press, 1985:3–37.
30. Thorn BE, Williams DA. Cognitive-behavioral management of chronic pain. In: VandeCreek L, Knapp S, Jackson TL, eds. Innovations in Clinical Practice: A Source Book. Sarasota: Professional Resource Press, 1993.
31. Morley S, Eccleston C, Williams A. Systematic review and meta-analysis of randomized controlled trials of cognitive behaviour therapy and behaviour therapy for chronic pain in adults, excluding headache. Pain 1999; 80(1–2):1–13.
32. Keefe FJ, Caldwell DS. Cognitive behavioral control of arthritis pain. Med Clin North Am 1997; 81(1):277–290.

33. Keefe FJ, Van HY. Cognitive-behavioral treatment of rheumatoid arthritis pain: maintaining treatment gains. Arthritis Care Res 1993; 6(4):213–222.
34. Keefe FJ, Caldwell DS, Williams DA, et al. Pain coping skills training in the management of osteoarthritic knee pain: a comparative study. Behav Ther 1990; 21:49–62.
35. Rossy LA, Buckelew SP, Dorr N, et al. A meta-analysis of fibromyalgia treatment interventions. Ann Behav Med 1999; 21(2):180–191.
36. Keefe FJ. Cognitive behavioral therapy for managing pain. Clin Psychol 1996; 49(3): 4–5.
37. N.I.H. Integration of behavioral and relaxation approaches into the treatment of chronic pain and insomnia. NIH technology assessment panel on integration of behavioral and relaxation approaches into the treatment of chronic pain and insomnia. J Am Med Assoc 1996; 276(4):313–318.
38. Lewinsohn PM. The behavioral study and treatment of depression. In: Hersen M, Eisler RM, Miller PM, eds. Progress in Behavior Modification. New York: Academic Press, 1975.
39. Lindstrom I, Ohlund C, Eek C, et al. The effect of graded activity on patients with subacute low back pain: a randomized prospective clinical study with an operant-conditioning behavioral approach. Phys Ther 1992; 72(4):279–290.
40. Gil KM, Ross SL, Keefe FJ. Behavioral treatment of chronic pain: four pain management protocols. In: France RD, Krishnan KRR, eds. Chronic Pain. New York: American Psychiatric Press, 1988.
41. Deale A, Chalder T, Marks I, et al. Cognitive behavior therapy for chronic fatigue syndrome: a randomized controlled trial. Am J Psychiatry 1997; 154(3):408–414.
42. Morin CM, Culbert JP, Schwartz SM. Nonpharmacological interventions for insomnia: a meta-analysis of treatment efficacy. Am J Psychiatry 1994; 151(8):1172–1180.
43. Affleck G, Tennen H, Urrows S, et al. Fibromyalgia and women's pursuit of personal goals: a daily process analysis. Health Psychol 1998; 17(1):40–47.
44. Affleck G, Urrows S, Tennen H, et al. Sequential daily relations of sleep, pain intensity, and attention to pain among women with fibromyalgia. Pain 1996; 68 (2–3):363–368.
45. Edinger JD, Wohlgemuth WK, Krystal AD, et al. Behavioral insomnia therapy for fibromyalgia patients: a randomized clinical trial. Arch Intern Med 2005; 165 (21):2527–2535.
46. Eccleston C, Crombez G. Attention and pain: merging behavioural and neuroscience investigations. Pain 2005; 113(1–2):7–8.
47. Eccleston C, Crombez G. Pain demands attention: a cognitive-affective model of the interruptive function of pain. Psychol Bull 1999; 125(3):356–366.
48. D'Zurilla TJ, Goldfried MR. Problem solving and behavior modification. J Abnorm Psychol 1971; 78(1):107–126.
49. Nezu AM, Nezu CM, Perri MG. Problem-Solving Therapy for Depression: Theory, Research and Clinical Guidelines. New York: Wiley & Sons, 1989.
50. Beck AT, Rush AJ, Shaw BF, et al. Cognitive Therapy and Depression. New York: The Guilford Press, 1979.
51. Goldfried MR, Davidson G. Clinical Behavioural Therapy. New York: Holt, Rinehart & Winston, 1976.
52. Gombeski WR Jr., Kramer K, Wilson T, et al. Women's Heart Advantage program: motivating rapid and assertive behavior. J Cardiovasc Manag 2002; 13(5):21–28.
53. Naylor MR, Keefe FJ, Brigidi B, et al. Therapeutic interactive voice response for chronic pain reduction and relapse prevention. Pain 2008; 134(3):335–345.
54. Lorig K, Feigenbaum P, Regan C, et al. A comparison of lay-taught and professional-taught arthritis self-management courses. J Rheumatol 1986; 13(4):763–767.
55. Tomkins S. Affect, Imagery, and Consciousness: The Positive Affects. New York: Springer, 1962.
56. Tomkins S. Affect, Imagery, and Consciousness: The Negative Affects. New York: Springer, 1963.
57. McClelland DC. Achievement and entrepreneurship: a longitudinal study. J Pers Soc Psychol 1965; 1:389–892.

58. McClelland DC. Power: The Inner Experience. New York: Irvingston-Halsted-Wiley, 1975.
59. White RW. Motivation reconsidered: the concept of competence. Psychol Rev 1959; 66:297–333.
60. Rotter JB. Social Learning and Clinical Psychology. Englewood Cliffs, NJ: Prentice Hall, 1954.
61. Rotter JB. Generalized expectancies for internal versus external control of reinforcement. Psychol Monogr 1966; 80:1–28.
62. Weiner B. An Attributional Theory of Motivation and Emotion. New York, NY: Springer-Verlag, 1986.
63. Bandura A, O'Leary A, Taylor CB, et al. Perceived self-efficacy and pain control: opioid and nonopioid mechanisms. J Pers Soc Psychol 1987; 53(3):563–571.
64. Lepper MR. Motivational considerations in the study of instruction. Cogn Instruct 1988; 5(4):289–309.
65. Kalleberg AL. Work values and job rewards: a theory of job satisfaction. Am Sociol Rev 2006; 42(1):124–143.
66. Linder JR. Understanding employee motivation. J Extension 1998; 36(3):1–8.
67. Jensen MP, Karoly P. Control beliefs, coping efforts, and adjustment to chronic pain. J Consult Clin Psychol 1991; 59(3):431–438.
68. Hersen M. Token economies in institutional settings. Historical, political, deprivation, ethical, and generalization issues. J Nerv Ment Dis 1976; 162(3):206–211.
69. Burckhardt CS. Nonpharmacologic management strategies in fibromyalgia. Rheum Dis Clin North Am 2002; 28(2):291–304.
70. Wallston KA, Wallston BS, DeVellis R. Development of the Multidimensional Health Locus of Control (MHLC) scales. Health Educ Monogr 1978; 6(2):160–170.
71. Coan RW. Personality variables associated with cigarette smoking. J Pers Soc Psychol 1973; 26:86–104.
72. Kaplan GD, Cowles L. Health locus of control and health value in the prediction of smoking reduction. Health Educ Monogr 1978; 6:129–137.
73. Balch P, Ross AW. Predicting success in weight reduction as a function of locus of control: a unidimensional and multidimensional approach. J Consult Clin Psychol 1975; 43:119.
74. Saltzer EB. Health locus of control and the intention to lose weight. Health Educ Monogr 1978; 6:118–127.
75. MacDonald AP. Internal-external locus of control and practice of birth control. Psychol Rep 1970; 27:206.
76. Dabbs JM, Kirscht JP. "Internal control" and the taking of influenza shots. Psychol Rep 1971; 28:959–962.
77. Findley MJ, Cooper HM. Locus of control and academic achievement: a literature review. J Pers Soc Psychol 1983; 44:419–427.
78. Anderman LH, Midgley C. Motivation and middle school students. In: Irwin JL, ed. What Current Research Says to the Middle Level Practitioner? Columbus, OH: National Middle School Association, 1997:41–48.
79. Burckhardt CS, Bjelle A. Perceived control: a comparison of women with fibromyalgia, rheumatoid arthritis, and systemic lupus erythematosus using a Swedish version of the Rheumatology Attitudes Index. Scand J Rheumatol 1996; 25(5): 300–306.
80. Gustafsson M, Gaston-Johansson F. Pain intensity and health locus of control: a comparison of patients with fibromyalgia syndrome and rheumatoid arthritis. Patient Educ Couns 1996; 29(2):179–188.
81. Pastor MA, Salas E, Lopez S, et al. Patients' beliefs about their lack of pain control in primary fibromyalgia syndrome. Br J Rheumatol 1993; 32(6):484–489.
82. Crisson JE, Keefe FJ. The relationship of locus of control to pain coping strategies and psychological distress in chronic pain patients. Pain 1988; 35(2):147–154.
83. Rudy TE, Kerns RD, Turk DC. Chronic pain and depression: toward a cognitive-behavioral mediation model. Pain 1988; 35(2):129–140.

84. Jensen MP, Turner JA, Romano JM, et al. Coping with chronic pain: a critical review of the literature. Pain 1991; 47(3):249–283.
85. Strong J, Ashton R, Cramond T, et al. Pain intensity, attitude and function in back pain patients. Aust Occup Ther J 1990; 37(4):179–183.
86. Gibson SJ, Helme RD. Cognitive factors and the experience of pain and suffering in older persons. Pain 2000; 85:375–383.
87. Lipchik GL, Milles K, Covington EC. The effects of multidisciplinary pain management treatment on locus of control and pain beliefs in chronic non-terminal pain. Clin J Pain 1993; 9(1):49–57.
88. Hagglund KJ, Haley WE, Reveille JD, et al. Predicting individual differences in pain and functional impairment among patients with rheumatoid arthritis. Arthritis Rheum 1989; 32:851–858.
89. Flor H, Turk DC. Chronic back pain and rheumatoid arthritis: predicting pain and disability from cognitive variables. J Behav Med 1988; 11(3):251–265.
90. Parker JC, Frank RG, Beck NC, et al. Pain management in rheumatoid arthritis patients. A cognitive-behavioral approach. Arthritis Rheum 1988; 31(5):593–601.
91. McCarberg B, Wolf J, Oliver K, et al. The relationship between health locus of control and well-being in fibromyalgia patients. J Pain 2002; 3(2):14.
92. Wittink H, Cohen LJ. The behavioral role of physical therapy in pain mangement. Curr Rev Pain 1998; 2:55–60.
93. Coughlin AM, Badura AS, Fleischer TD, et al. Multidisciplinary treatment of chronic pain patients: its efficacy in changing patient locus of control. Arch Phys Med Rehabil 2000; 81:739–740.
94. Prochaska JO, DiClemente CC. Stages and processes of self-change of smoking: toward an integrative model of change. J Consult Clin Psychol 1983; 51(3):390–395.
95. Prochaska JO, DiClemente CC, Velicer WF, et al. Standardized, individualized, interactive, and personalized self-help programs for smoking cessation. Health Psychol 1993; 12(5):399–405.
96. Kerns RD, Rosenberg R, Jamison RN, et al. Readiness to adopt a self-management approach to chronic pain: the Pain Stages of Change Questionnaire (PSOCQ). Pain 1997; 72(1–2):227–234.
97. Jones KD, Burckhardt CS, Bennett JA. Motivational interviewing may encourage exercise in persons with fibromyalgia by enhancing self-efficacy. Arthritis Rheum 2004; 51(5):864–867.
98. Kersten L. Changes in self-concept during pulmonary rehabilitation, Part 1. Heart Lung 1990; 19(5 pt 1):456–462.

Fibromyalgia Management for the Primary Care Provider

Bill H. McCarberg

Chronic Pain Management Program, Kaiser Permanente San Diego, and University of California, San Diego, California, U.S.A.

INTRODUCTION

National statistics confirm what every primary care provider has always suspected—pain is the most common reason that patients seek medical care. It accounts for up to 80% of visits to physicians' offices in the United States (1,2), and recent surveys suggest that as many as 75 to 105 million Americans experience pain daily or intermittently (3–5). In most cases, both the patient and the physician understand the underlying disease process—for instance, pharyngitis, gastroenteritis, or migraine headache—and prescribed treatments are effective in resolving the painful symptom. When pain is persistent, and the underlying condition cannot be "cured" even with specialty care, medical management of the patient becomes difficult. This is especially true for patients with fibromyalgia (FM).

FM abounds with uncertainties. Pathophysiology is uncertain, etiology is uncertain, natural course in a patient is uncertain. Many experts question the existence of the disease making the diagnosis itself uncertain. FM is not a disease and it is politically incorrect to call it a syndrome, making the name uncertain. There are very few proven effective management strategies but many home-grown options claiming cure that the treatment is uncertain. Primary care providers are comfortable dealing with uncertainty in medicine. However this degree of uncertainty makes every medical decision difficult. The lack of a cure and the effect of the disease on the patient's physical and emotional status contribute to making FM one of the most difficult conditions seen in primary care practices.

In a recent survey of internists, only 34% reported feeling comfortable with their abilities to manage a patient with chronic pain (2). Often the discomfort felt by physicians is due, in part, to a lack of understanding of pain assessment techniques and limited knowledge of available pain therapies. In the case of FM, skepticism about the diagnosis may compound the physician's discomfort and hamper his or her ability to provide the compassion and support that is a hallmark of primary care.

Despite continued efforts to improve pain management in primary care, current practice is suboptimal at best (6,7). Patients report that their physicians do not ask about pain, that they are afraid to report pain, and that treatment is not offered. Even with recent advances in pain research, pharmaceuticals, complementary and alternative therapies, and intervention techniques, undertreatment of chronic pain is considered pandemic. The solution lies with primary care providers.

As the patient's "medical home," the primary care setting is uniquely suited to provide medical management for patients with FM. Primary care providers develop longitudinal relationships with patients and are experienced in providing comfort and disease management for conditions that have no cure. They are accustomed to maintaining a nonjudgmental attitude while persuading patients to improve their health through exercise, diet, stress management, appropriate medications, and disease monitoring—and they are equally accustomed to patient's nonadherence. The first step in treating FM is to set aside any personal biases and beliefs about the condition and focus on the patient.

PRIMARY CARE CHALLENGES IN PAIN MANAGEMENT
Many barriers to the management of pain are well documented in this text and others, with obstacles relating to the medical system, providers, patients, and regulatory and governmental agencies as shown in Table 1.

While these barriers are substantial, other obstacles that are unique to primary care make pain management challenging even for the well-trained, conscientious provider.

The Shrinking Office Visit
Of all the barriers encountered by primary care, lack of sufficient time is the most problematic. Even the most complex medical problem can be evaluated and treated given the luxury of unlimited time. Without time constraints, complete histories, questionnaires, routine preventive care, physical exams, follow-up care for existing conditions, consultations, and orders for testing and imaging can be accommodated. In reality, the steady increases in external requirements (i.e., payers, regulatory organizations) and healthcare costs coupled with cuts in reimbursement have forced primary care providers to do more with fewer resources—in less time. As more patients schedule in shorter visits to compensate for reduced visit reimbursement rates, nonroutine problems become more challenging. Patients with uncertain diagnoses and overlaying psychosocial issues consume precious office time. Suffering from continued pain and depression over time, these patients are often dissatisfied and angry about the failure of medical treatment.

Multiple problems must be addressed in the relatively brief primary care office encounter. In addition to the patient's complaints of pain, insomnia, depression, and family stress, the physician needs to monitor other chronic

TABLE 1 Barriers to Pain Appropriate Pain Management[a]

Medical system	Access to medical care	Access to specialists	Denied coverage of medication or procedures	Denied coverage of CAM therapy[a]	Preauthorization requirements
Patient	Poor lifestyle choices	Fear to accept proven treatment	Expectation of cure	Stigma of psychiatric care	Beliefs about aging
Providers	Time pressure	Lack of knowledge	Bias toward treatment	Nialistic care	Beliefs about pain and aging
Regulatory and governmental agencies	Lack of medicare reimbursement	Oversight of opioid prescribing			

[a]American Pain Society. Guideline for the Management of Pain in Osteoarthritis, Rhyematoid Arthritis and Juvenile Chronic Arthritis. 2nd ed. Glenview, IL: American Pain Society, 2002.

conditions (e.g., diabetes, hypertension), attend to screenings and immunizations, refill prescriptions, and review laboratory reports. Questions from staff, telephone calls from other patients, and walk-in or add-on appointments also encroach on time. It should come as no surprise that some specialists believe that pain patients receive substandard care from primary care physicians because of poor documentation or inadequate follow-up.

As patients gain more knowledge, they develop greater expectations that further complicate pain management. Patients exposed to media events, consumer advertising, and health information sites on the Internet often expect more in the way of testing, referrals, treatment, and cures. Conditions such as FM require complicated drug combinations in a trial and error approach, with frequent visits and follow-up to determine adequacy of treatment. Additional visits become more difficult with already full schedules and large patient loads.

Guidelines

It is easy to work efficiently when the evaluation process and optimal treatment are clear-cut. Even a complex condition like diabetes has become less daunting to treat with well-established guidelines to follow when managing patients. In medical training all providers learn the important historical questions, the in-office examination, and the required treatment. Even without memory aids or consultation, every primary care provider knows the stepwise process of care for a diabetic patient—a process that is standardized throughout the country. Such a guideline-based approach facilitates comprehensive care in a brief office visit.

Although guidelines exist for FM[b], they have not been widely distributed and are largely unknown to primary care[c] in general. These guidelines may not be used by local pain experts, leading less experienced providers to question their credibility. Education can always help remedy a lack of knowledge, but there are practical issues involved in diagnosing and treating FM.

Outcomes

Experiencing a successful outcome leads the provider to continuing the treatment. When a diabetic patient lowers the HgA_1C, the treatment effort is worthwhile and the success is repeated. What is the measurable outcome in chronic pain? Pain scores can be measured, but pain frequently does not improve. An improved functional outcome is also important, but how do you measure increased function? In diabetes, hypertension, congestive heart failure, and chronic obstructive pulmonary disease there is a known, easily understood, and measurable outcome. In chronic pain, this is not taught and is frequently difficult to determine.

Nonadherence

Nonadherence is common in primary care and providers acknowledge the difficulty in persuading a patient to change a longstanding behavior to one that is medically prudent. If a patient's $HgbA_1C$ does not improve, we do not get

[b]American Pain Society. Guidelines for the Management of Fibromyalgia Syndrome Pain in Adults and Children. Glenview, IL: American Pain Society, 2005.
[c]McCarberg, B. Impact of guidelines on healthcare from the patient and payor perspective: example of the American Pain Society Guidelines. Dis Manag Health Outcome 2004; 12(1):73–79.

angry or accuse the patient but recommend diet and exercise and continue following the patient. If our patient does not stop smoking, we continue to treat the patient but persist in suggesting a smoking cessation program.

When a patient does not adhere to pain treatment, especially when this treatment involves opioid therapy, we have a different reaction. Patient's non-adherence can lead to risk for the provider in the form of regulatory scrutiny or criminal investigation. In pain management, patient's nonadherence generates a higher level of discomfort for the treating physician and often leads to a desire to stop caring for the patient.

Advocacy Vs. Adversarial Relationship

As a rule, primary care providers are patients' strongest advocates. Primary care providers help patients negotiate the complex healthcare system, interact on their behalf with insurers for treatment options, referrals, and hospital care. The bond developed through longstanding relationships helps in this advocacy through knowledge of how the patient functions.

Pain management is an area where advocacy can turn abruptly into an adversarial relationship. Patients suffering from FM often want things that are not in their best interest—time off work or disability, handicapped parking forms, repeated expensive diagnostic procedures, and unproven/dangerous treatments—and resist. When the mutual trust and bond that usually characterize provider-patient interactions is replaced with arguments, resentment, and misunderstandings, the provider begins to dread seeing the patient. In turn, the chronic pain patient is left feeling frustrated and helpless.

Chronic Illness and Disease Management

Most chronic illness is handled in primary care (Table 2). Despite the many obstacles, primary care is still the best provider to care for the FM patient.

As in all chronic pain conditions, patients with FM often display a variety of related symptoms such as fatigue, sleep disorders, deconditioning, psychological distress, and cognitive dysfunction. Patients with FM often experience stresses in every sphere of life—work, social, family, leisure activities—resulting in decreased quality of life. The pervasive nature of the condition makes FM amenable to disease management, a holistic, multidisciplinary approach that includes pharmacological and nonpharmacological strategies as well as patient education, acceptance, and self-help skills aimed at helping patients deal with their compromised quality of life.

The primary care provider's long-term relationship with and knowledge of patient—how the patient reacts to disease, stress, injury, loss, cancer—is

TABLE 2 Chronic Medical Conditions Treated in Primary Care

Condition	Primary care (%)	Others (%)
ASCVD	86	14
Stroke	91	9
Hypertension	92	8
Diabetes	90	10
Chronic obstructive lung disease	89	11
Asthma	94	6

Source: From Ref. (8).

extraordinarily valuable. Such understanding enables the primary care provider to take account of the specific coping strategies of each patient, an essential ingredient for effective disease management.

Patients with FM are distributed throughout the United States, many in areas isolated from advanced medical care. Given the lack of pain specialists— there are only 6000 doctors (9) with boards in pain medicine and a majority of these are in large urban areas—the only medical community capable of caring for this population is primary care. Primary care has shown itself capable of managing all other complex, chronic conditions in exemplary fashion. It is fitting that primary care leads the way in managing the chronic pain condition.

Practical Pain Management

Given the many barriers to care, primary care providers need a practical approach to managing FM. Time considerations, perhaps the greatest challenge, will benefit from the further development and dissemination of diagnostic and treatment guidelines. The following are practical steps that the primary care provider can take to streamline the management of FM pain in a busy office practice.

Validation

Validating the patient—asking the patient what he or she wants—can streamline the visit. Asking the patient, "What do you think I can do to help your pain?" opens a dialog about expectations and responsibilities while streamlining the visit. Concerns that the patient will request something we cannot deliver such as total pain relief, or another magnetic resonance imaging, or more opioids are largely unfounded.

There is concern that giving the patient the diagnosis may enable unhealthy, sick-role behavior. In a study of patients with FM syndrome, providing a diagnosis resulted in the patient making fewer visits to the physician's office and becoming more empowered and proactive (e.g., more likely to investigate self-help techniques) (10).

Assessment Tools

Chronic pain always starts as an acute pain episode. Even a chronic illness like FM starts with a new muscle ache, fatigue, or sleep disorder. It can take months before the correct diagnosis is elucidated and the care provider knows that he or she is facing a long-term problem that can be difficult to manage. At this point, the care provider's attention should focus on disease management—that is, symptom improvement rather than multiple interventions and cure.

How can this evaluation be done in a short office visit? Evaluation needs to focus on the desired outcome of pain reduction, function improvement, and identification and management of comorbidities. While this evaluation can take several visits, handouts and questionnaires can be useful in streamlining the process.

Try giving the patient forms to complete at home to measure pain, function, depression, and anxiety. Many patients like having the ability to describe issues in greater detail than they would during a brief office visit. Follow-up visit is then designed to review the results. The handouts direct the follow-up visit on important outcome variables: pain and function. The patient knows what outcomes are important and what each subsequent visit will address.

Patients frequently resist discussing depression because they equate depression with an unreal pain, a complaint that is "all in my head." As a medical provider, one knows that depression and pain are often comorbid illnesses, and that treating depression improves quality of life. Once a patient self-reports anxiety or depression on a questionnaire, the medical provider has the information on a form providing the diagnosis. This is not a value judgment. The medical provider is not trying to disregard or depreciate the pain. The form is filled out by the patient and the discussion becomes easier. Thus, treating these comorbidities takes less time.

Plan of Action

As in other chronic illnesses, patient participation and adherence to treatment recommendations predict better outcomes. FM affects many life activities and, in turn, quality of life. Goal-setting discussions direct the patient to improved activity and a targeted outcome; for instance, if the patient wants and agrees to walk 10 minutes a day or work in the garden, either of these might serve as a goal to track at each visit. As patients begin to anticipate the questions the physician will ask about their goals, visits will become more streamlined and will focus on a functional outcome.

Once the physician evaluates the patient and the treatment has been initiated, follow-up of the patient with FM in a 15-minute visit may seem a challenge. In reality, follow-up does not take a great deal of time if the physician keeps the focus on the desired outcome. Consider all that one can accomplish in the same 15 minutes when following a patient with diabetes: asking about diet, exercise, foot numbness, vision, and home glucose monitoring; and adjusting treatment based on all the information received. The problem with a follow-up visit for FM is that the physician often does not know what to follow, what to ask, and what variables to track. The appointment becomes a forum for the patient's complaints about pain, disability, and poor quality of life—and time for effective patient management is constrained.

When prescribing opioids for pain management, primary care physicians are faced with scenarios that depict potential addiction in patients: early refills, lost or stolen medication, borrowed medication, and failed urine drug tests. Documentation must be quick yet complete. The four A's of treatment success enable the primary care physician to concentrate on essential outcomes to the patient's overall quality of life and save time (11).

A_1—analgesia or pain score.

A_2—activities of daily living or functional outcome that is meaningful to the patient. In this setting the goal-setting discussion accomplishes this target.

A_3—adverse events. Anticipating and soliciting side effects from treatment allows for adverse event management rather than discarding effective pain treatment.

A_4—aberrant behavior. Has a behavior occurred that is worrisome such as requests for early refills? What does this behavior mean and how will you address it?

MOTIVATING BEHAVIOR CHANGE IN PATIENTS WITH FM

Successful management of chronic pain is much more dependent on what the patient does than on what the physician does to the patient. The issue becomes one of patient's readiness to accept responsibility and to adopt a self-management approach. This represents a role reversal for the physician whose task is not to treat but to understand and motivate patients for self-management.

Primary care physicians' unique relationships with patients can be the key to motivating patients to change. A patient-centered approach used in all chronic illnesses emphasizes the patient's perspective when making treatment recommendations. What the diabetic believes about his or her illness leads to strategies to motivate behavior. The goals of a patient-centered approach are to address the patient's concerns, enhance a collaborative relationship, provide information that the patient is ready to hear, refocus the visit from making treatment recommendations to supporting the patient's self-care, and foster increased patient control of decision-making and responsibility for self-care. This approach is practiced daily in primary care and lends itself to the management of FM as well.

CONCLUSION

Even though patients with a sympathetic provider to help them with chronic pain are some of the most appreciative, primary care physicians are unenthusiastic when faced with treating patients with FM. These complex patients are rarely cured, make little progress toward normal life functioning, and often have psychosocial issues that further complicate management. There is never enough time to adequately follow-up pain patients. At the same time, the primary care provider is uniquely suited to dealing with chronic problems through short, focused visits and with the benefit of a longitudinal experience with patients. Primary care providers are experienced in dealing with other difficult, complex care issues and can translate this expertise into caring for patients with FM.

REFERENCES

1. Harstall C. How prevalent is chronic pain? Pain Clin Updat 2003; 10:1–4.
2. O'Rorke JE, Chen I, Genao I, et al. Physicians' comfort in caring for patients with chronic nonmalignant pain. Am J Med Sci 2007; 333:93–100.
3. Gallup, Inc. Pain in America: highlights from a Gallup survey. June 9, 1999.
4. Bostrom BM, Ramberg T, Davis BD, et al. Survey of post-operative patients' pain management. J Nurs Manag 1997; 5:341–349.
5. Dworkin R, Backonja M, Rowbotham M, et al. Advances in neuropathic pain: diagnosis, mechanisms, and treatment recommendations. Arch Neurol 2003; 60:1524–1534.
6. Dahlman G-B, Dykes A-K, Elander G. Patients' evaluation of pain and nurses' management of analgesics after surgery. The effect of a study day on the subject of pain for nurses working at the thorax surgery department. J Adv Nurs 1999; 30: 866–874.
7. Drayer R, Henderson J, Reidenberg M. Barriers to better pain control in hospitalized patient. J Pain Symptom Manage 1999; 17:434–440.
8. Ann Fam Med 2004; 2(suppl 1).
9. Estimate of diplomates certified in pain from the American Board of Pain Medicine and American Board of Anesthesiology.
10. White KP, Nielson WR, Harth M, et al. Does the label "fibromyalgia" alter health status, function, and health service utilization? A prospective, within-group comparison in a community cohort of adults with chronic widespread pain. Arthritis Rheum 2002; 47:260–265.
11. Passik SD, Weinreb HJ. Managing chronic nonmalignant pain: overcoming obstacles to the use of opioids. Adv Ther 2000; 17(2):70–83.

Index

Acetominophen, 74
Acetyl-L-carnitine (LAC), 49
Acquired drives, in motivation theories, 142
Acupuncture, 42–44
Adaptive coping strategies, 95
Aerobic exercise, 128–131, 133
Affective spectrum disorder, 4
Aldolase, 30
Alpha-2-delta ligands, 68–69, 71–72
α-intrusions, 16
American College of Rheumatology (ACR), criteria for fibromyalgia, 2–4, 17, 56, 90, 104, 120
Amitriptyline, 13, 59
Anger, 91–92
Ankylosing spondylitis, 6
Anti-cyclic citrullinated peptide (anti-CCP), 33
Antidepressant therapy, 111
Anti-inflammatory medications, 74
Antinuclear antibody (ANA), 30
Anxiety, 88–90
  disorders, 16
Arteritis
  giant cell, 28–29
  temporal, 28–29
Arthralgias, 29
Arthritis Foundation based education program (FSCH), 50
Asthma, 81
Autoimmune inflammatory disorders, 28–30
Avoidance behavior, 89

Balneotherapy, 44, 130
Behavioral coping strategies, 95
Behavioral strategies for improving sleep and cognition, 139. *See also* Sleep in FM
Benzodiazepines, 72
Biochemical abnormalities, 15
Biofeedback, 47

Biological motives and primary affects, in motivation theories, 141–142
Body mass index (BMI), 48–49

Calcitonin gene-related peptide (CGRP), 11–12
Catastrophizing, 94–96
Cerebrospinal fluid (CSF) enkephalins, 11
Children with FM, exercise for, 133
Chronic fatigue syndrome (CFS), 136
Chronic illness and disease management, 155–156
Chronic pain
  angry feelings and, 91
  anxiety and, 88–90
  depression and, 90
  hypervigilance model, 95–96
  operant conditioning to, 85–87
  taxonomy of, 96
Chronic widespread pain (CWP), 2–5, 7, 136
Citalopram, 66
Classical conditioning, 84–85
Cognitive and psychological (CP) symptoms, of FM, 97–98
Cognitive behavioral therapy (CBT), 46–47
  barriers in implementing behavioral changes, 141
  delivery of, 140–141
  for fibromyalgia, 137–140
  skill sets common to FM, 137–140
    behavioral strategies for improving sleep and cognition, 139
    cognitive restructuring, 139–140
    communication skills training, 140
    graded activation, 138–139
    pleasant activity scheduling, 138–139
    problem-solving strategies, 139–140
    relaxation response, 137–138
Cognitive-interpretive processes, 89
Cognitive-perceptual processes, 89
Cognitive restructuring techniques, 139–140
Cold stimuli, 10

159

For Product Safety Concerns and Information please contact our
EU representative GPSR@taylorandfrancis.com Taylor & Francis
Verlag GmbH, Kaufingerstraße 24, 80331 München, Germany